The NEW NATURAL

YOUR ULTIMATE GUIDE TO CUTTING-EDGE AGE REVERSAL

Neil Sadick, MD

with Samantha Marshall and Adam Dinkes

RODALE.

© 2011 by Sadick Dermatology

Photographs © 2011 by Sadick Research Group

Rodale books may be purchased for business or promotional use or for special sales. For information, please write to:

Special Markets Department, Rodale, Inc., 733 Third Avenue, New York, NY 10017

Printed in the United States of America

Rodale Inc. makes every effort to use acid-free ♾, recycled paper ♻.

Illustrations by Alyssa Bieler and Karen Kuchar

Book design by Rich Kershner

Library of Congress Cataloging-in-Publication Data
Sadick, Neil S.
    The new natural : your ultimate guide to cutting-edge age reversal / Neal Sadick, with Samantha Marshall and Adam Dinkes.
        p.   cm.
    Includes index.
    ISBN 978–1–60961–125–5 hardcover
    1. Skin—Care and hygiene.   2. Rejuvenation.   3. Beauty, Personal.   I. Marshall, Samantha   II. Dinkes, Adam.   III. Title.
    RL87.S23   2011
    646.7`26—dc22   2011010325

Distributed to the trade by Macmillan

2 4 6 8 10 9 7 5 3 1 hardcover

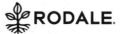

We inspire and enable people to improve their lives and the world around them.
www.rodalebooks.com

The
NEW
NATURAL

To my father, Harry, for his unwavering support, and to Sydney, my beautiful daughter, whose wisdom is beyond her years and who inspires me every day.

Let the beauty of what we love be what we do.
—Rumi

CONTENTS

PART III
REVERSE
(Ages 40 to 80 . . .)

WHAT IS POSSIBLE NOW

Ever look in the mirror and wish your skin were tighter or more youthful looking? Ever wish you could replace lost volume in your cheeks? Ever dream of eliminating acne scars or those dark circles under your eyes? Ever fantasize about melting, freezing, or sonically blasting your love handles or potbelly into oblivion? Well, you can! The last few years have seen a giant leap in the advancement of revolutionary cosmetic anti-aging procedures, and these beauty treatments and technologies are being tested for safety and efficacy in my offices as we speak. Ever wish there was some cream or serum that could thicken and tighten your skin, even help you stimulate new hair growth? Through stem cells and other forms of cell therapy, it's already happening, and in the coming years, further advancements will utterly transform the way we look at aging and at beauty.

Youth is a constant work in progress. But the good news is that there has been exponential progress in the tools and science that can address every aspect of visible aging, whether it's wrinkles, sagging, volume loss, hair loss, veins, discoloration, or stubborn pockets of body fat that are even harder to eliminate the older we get. What technology can do today, and the results it will be able to achieve tomorrow, is nothing short of miraculous.

My own discoveries in anti-aging and cosmetic treatments stem from my fascination with technology and science. Many of the treatments we use for aesthetic purposes today started out as protocols for medical conditions. Botox, for example, was used to alleviate muscle spasms; lasers were developed to help stroke patients with facial paralysis; certain fillers were used to improve quality of life in AIDS patients suffering from facial wasting. But the more I studied how these treatments and technologies worked, the more potential I saw for skin health and beauty. Figuring out exactly how light sources and sound waves interact at different levels of the skin's surface, heating and manipulating the structure of the cells, has opened up a world of possibilities beyond the traditional surgeon's knife.

We are changing the paradigm of age prevention and reversal. It's no longer about having a face-lift. In fact, you may never have to go under the knife to look like your best version of yourself. There is a non-invasive revolution taking place, even in the field of plastic surgery. Scalpels are out; lasers and tiny cannulas are in. We are moving away from the artificial, surgical look. The technology has evolved to the point where you can look amazing at any age, with minimal downtime and almost no risk of side effects. You won't have to hide your age, because with so many new technologies to help you age gracefully, 40, 50, 60, and 70 are going to look great on you. And perfectly . . . natural.

I'm probably a lot like you. I'll do whatever it takes to maintain my youth, as long as it doesn't involve too much pain or dramatically change the way I look. Very few of my patients have had face-lifts because they know they are not necessary if they take proper care of their skin. It doesn't matter if they have good genes or what their particular skin type happens to be. If you are fair-skinned, you don't have to accept wrinkles, freckles, discoloration, or any other signs of premature aging. The palest among us *can* look like Julianne Moore. It takes work. These patients take meticulous care of their skin, maintaining its elasticity and texture using only the best science-backed topical creams and turning to laser and radio-frequency technology, Botox and fillers, to stay on top of wrinkles and pigment as they occur. I'm proud to say that the women who come through my practice almost never look "done." Instead, they are living proof that it *is* possible to regenerate the skin . . . to restore youthful elasticity . . . to eliminate sagging . . . to eradicate deep wrinkles . . . to bring back the face that is the real you without resorting to traditional surgery.

This is not about looking perfect. The men and women I treat have no interest in looking as though they belong in Madame Tussaud's wax museum. They enjoy having facial expressions. Instead, the goal is to generate and maintain a skin texture that is youthful, healthy, and smooth. The color and tone are even; the pores are virtually invisible. By the time they reach their sixth decade, they don't have the telltale eye bags or sagging jowls. They have been able to slow the march of time by using the most advanced cosmeceuticals and injectable fillers to stimulate their own collagen and strengthen the overall structure of their skin cells. They use every advantage at my disposal—whether it's at the end of a needle or a laser—to get that glow of youth.

There's no single trick to looking younger than your real age. It should be a natural rejuvenation over time, using safe technology and scientifically tested topical solutions. As you would a vintage car, you can keep your exterior in mint condition with subtle detailing and continual maintenance.

In this book, I'll give you the same comprehensive menu of options for maintaining youth that I offer my patients: based on real, legitimate science. I do not promise instant gratification, the latest fads, or quick fixes. Plenty of skin doctors will boast, "Younger skin in 8 weeks" (or "5 minutes, 5 weeks"). But these solutions are deceptive. Even a face-lift isn't one-stop shopping. The prevailing wisdom is that a face-lift will ultimately be cheaper than multiple non-invasive treatments over a lifetime, and by the numbers that's perfectly true. But a scalpel doesn't cure age spots or build volume. And after another

10 years most people need a second face-lift. Then comes the third nip and tuck. No matter how brilliant your surgeon might be, after a few too many surgeries your face will be pulled back so tight that you might not be able to blink. And there's no going back. You can't replace skin that's already been removed. That "done" look can never be undone.

There's tremendous confusion out there when it comes to age reversal. Scientific advancements have reached a critical mass, but patients aren't getting the information they need from existing books or the media. Industry jargon is all over the place, and new skin care products making inflated claims of efficacy are piling up on the shelves. We all hear about the new products and gadgets, but no one is emphasizing *how* they should be used, and the results can be disastrous. It's time to cut through the clutter. You deserve to know exactly what techniques, formulations, and technologies give the best results in a particular scenario.

It starts with solid, research-based science. I've been a practicing dermatologist since the 1980s, and what technology can do today would have sounded like the stuff of science fiction back then. If I went back to the time I first opened my practice and told colleagues it was possible to remove fat nonsurgically, they'd laugh and call me crazy. But now patients are losing inches and reshaping their legs, hips, and stomachs without going under the knife. Even when I first suggested more than a decade ago that lasers could be used for hair removal and certain skin conditions, I was accused of being a mad scientist. But today the laser and light sources I helped develop have blossomed into a multibillion-dollar global industry.

There's nothing I recommend in this book that I haven't tried on myself or my very willing research and clinical staff. We don't hype what hasn't been thoroughly researched and proven for safety and results. I am on a constant quest to make sure the science of eternal youth is truly effective and long lasting, and it is my mission to deliver the tools of age reversal to everyone. Youth should not be the privilege of just the wealthy or famous. There are new mass-market lotions and creams that can protect and rejuvenate the skin and reverse the signs of aging just as effectively as the most expensive brands. I will tell you which of these products are best and which will soon see further improvements and become even more affordable. I will show you little tricks you can do to prolong the effects of more expensive in-office treatments and introduce you to the new generations of at-home devices that can achieve wonders for your appearance.

You should also know that no single technology offers the ultimate magic bullet. Each and every age reversal program should be multifaceted and tailored to each patient. Your individual beauty deserves more than a one-size-fits-all solution. And looking and feeling your best goes hand in hand with maintaining your internal health. When my patients are happy with their appearance, they tend to take better care of themselves. They dress better, work out more, socialize more, and walk through life with confidence.

It's a natural impulse to want to do everything you can to maintain a healthy, youthful appearance. But that look has nothing to do with the wind-tunnel effect the world has come to associate with cosmetic procedures and plastic surgery. A 50-year-old woman who is trying to look 25 does not look either healthy or youthful. What we are striving for here is anything but plastic. It's not fake. It's not overdone. It's the New Natural.

AUTHOR'S NOTE

Unless otherwise stated, names and identifying details of patients have been changed to protect doctor-patient confidentiality. All examples are based on real cases and composites.

PART I

PREVENT

(Ages 0 to 80)

CHAPTER ONE

THE NATURAL AESTHETIC

NOBODY IS PERFECT

Ann couldn't recognize herself anymore. After multiple cosmetic procedures, including a brow-lift, a neck-lift, and a nose job, she was starting to get that alien plastic look, and she was distraught. The 55-year-old housewife from Long Island had so much filler in her cheeks that she looked as if she had balloons under her eyes, her lips—overly plumped with silicone—resembled those of a platypus, and their disproportion made the rest of her features look as if they didn't belong on her face. When Ann showed me a picture of how she looked before she had all that work done, I noticed that she had once been a stunningly beautiful woman. She had a few lines and folds, and a little sagging around the jowls, but nothing that would have required the drastic surgical intervention she had endured over the years.

Many aging women just like Ann have bought into the myth that cosmetic surgery can turn them back into their younger selves, and the results can be disastrous. And every time they try to improve upon the first bad job, it just gets worse. That's when they come to see me.

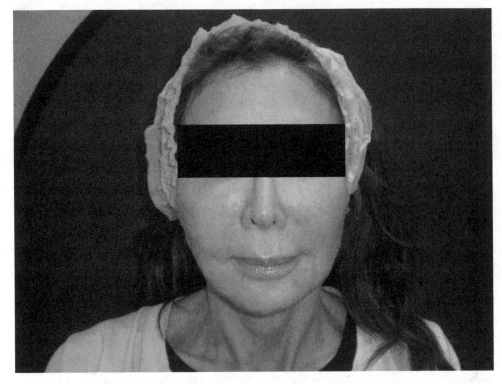

The above patient has had multiple treatments and surgeries, resulting in an unnatural look: overfilled mid-cheeks, uneven lips, and an overly taut, pulled appearance from excessive brow and face lifts.

While I couldn't get Ann completely back to the pre-surgical look she was born with, I could clear up some of her damage with a few fine-tuned procedures (all of which I will discuss in more detail throughout the book). Luckily, the filler in her cheeks was Restylane, which has an antidote. After I toned down that puffy chipmunk look, she already looked much better and more natural. But there were still several pull marks on the side of her face from the lifts, so I treated her with a laser resurfacing procedure, which softened the lines and greatly improved the overall texture of her skin. A few weeks later, I added Sculptra—a volumizing filler—deep below the skin's surface, to correct the architecture of her face as much as I could and to build a more natural plumpness around her cheeks. The lips were another matter. The silicone could be removed only with a painful surgical procedure, and the resulting scarring could be worse than what she already had. I referred her to a plastic surgeon I trusted and encouraged her to weigh the pros and cons of yet another potentially risky surgery.

LESS IS MORE

The anti-aging treatments I discuss in this book are not meant to turn you into a totally different person. They are designed to correct marks of aging gradually and gently as they occur so that you can maintain your natural looks and always look gorgeous, young, and healthy—*for your decade.* Don't make Ann's mistake and try to look unrealistically younger.

Appreciate your unique beauty and do everything you can to protect what you already have. Instead of seeking the surgical quick fix, focus on the new paradigm for age prevention and reversal: cell turnover, or the shedding of dead skin cells to make way for younger cells and improve the texture of your skin's surface and stimulation of collagen, a major component of connective tissue. Collagen is basically protein, made up of amino acids strung together like long chains of linked building blocks, and it is the foundation that gives your skin its support and thickness. The more collagen you have, the tighter the skin and the more you can fight against gravitational pull. In later chapters, I will discuss many ways you can put your skin to work for you. Maintaining a natural, youthful look is not about cutting and removing skin as you would in a face-lift. Instead, the focus should be on volume repletion for thick, plump, youthful skin.

Before I launch into the various anti-aging options you might want to consider at different stages in life, you should know that I am biased. Everything I stand for is about reversing the past trends that have distorted our perceptions of human beauty and caused lifelong damage to patients like Ann. Ninety percent of the time I advocate against plastic or cosmetic surgery, but I am not saying never. I am a board-certified cosmetic surgeon and I do occasionally perform surgical procedures, but for most of my patients, I just don't feel that cutting and removing skin and fat tissue are necessary.

HOW MUCH IS TOO MUCH?

Doctors and patients have lost sight of what's natural when it comes to the aesthetics of cosmetic enhancement and age reversal. Young actresses are distorting their features with fillers to create pouts like a pair of sausages. It's not sexy, it's comical. And it doesn't look real. Women are getting child-like button noses that don't fit their faces. Women and men are getting brow-lifts that pull their faces up so high, they look permanently surprised. When I see these patients, I immediately think of Howdy Doody. Other patients are freezing their faces into perfect Botox masks and going crazy with injectable fillers and implants for a lumpy, cartoonish effect.

People generally know when someone has had too much done—whether it's a nip and tuck or filler. We've all seen the celebrities with cosmetic procedure disasters. They're under enough public scrutiny, so I am not going to add my voice to the choir by naming names. All you have to do is pick up a tabloid at the supermarket checkout for the latest in the list of top 10 worst makeovers. But the trick is knowing when you are going too far on your *own* path to age reversal. It's hard for us to see ourselves as others do. We may focus on a flaw that we think needs to be corrected where the rest of the world sees nothing. A doctor can guide us, and even opt to refuse a procedure, but patients can always find someone less scrupulous who is willing to give them what they believe they need.

Eyes, lips, nose, cheeks—these are all features that can throw off the proportions of the rest of the face. Lips are the most common problem area, which is why I always urge patients to leave them alone. But it's all

KEEP IT REAL!

◆ Set your skin up for success with proper prevention: sunblocks, antioxidants, cosmeceuticals, and proactive skin care.

◆ Choose a practitioner with aesthetic goals that match yours—if a doctor is known for one look, it's not likely that you will get something different.

◆ Build good anti-aging practices now to avoid drastic surgical measures later.

too easy to overfill other areas of the face as well. Instead of looking rested and refreshed, a patient who goes too far looks puffy, even lumpy. So manage your own expectations and decide what you are really going for when you step into that doctor's office. Bring in a picture of yourself looking your best 5 to 10 years ago to give the doctor a visual guide. Much depends on the aesthetic sense of your dermatologist or plastic surgeon. Make sure their artistic instincts lean toward the subtle. Ask to see as many before and after pictures as you can. That is your right as a patient. The rest is up to you.

You know you are in good shape when your friends have no idea you've gotten work done. They think you look great and assume it's because you've spent the last month at the spa. They ask you where you went on vacation. But if they starting asking you who did your nose, or your eyes, or your cheek implants, it's a bad sign. And if they say nothing because they are too embarrassed to draw attention to the elephant in the room, it's even worse.

THE NEW NATURAL

Recently there's been a backlash to this quest for inhuman perfection. Hollywood actresses who have had too much surgery are losing roles. Casting directors are eschewing the frozen foreheads in favor of women who can move their faces and show emotion. They're giving the juicy parts to actresses from outside of Los Angeles, and even outside of America, where the plastic surgery craze hasn't gone as far and most women in show business still have their original noses and lips.

One of the best examples of that rare actress who has aged gracefully is Betty White. While she has been tweaked over the years, she still looks age appropriate, and her recent comeback is a clear sign that we are appreciating people with a more natural, realistic appearance.

This new natural look is what discerning men and women are now asking for when they come to my office. They want a combination of volume, elasticity, and smooth, supple skin with few (if any) wrinkles. And *no* surgery! Take my patient Barbara, for example. When she first breezed into my office, I could tell she'd taken great care of herself over the years. She was one of those perfectly groomed, elegant women you often see out shopping or walking their poodles on Madison Avenue. A nonsmoker who avoided the sun and rarely drank, she had very few wrinkles for a woman who was probably in her mid- to late fifties. But she wasn't happy.

"Doc, I need a pick-me-up. I'm starting to look like somebody's mother. I'm not ready for that."

I asked her: "Barbara, exactly what is it you are hoping to achieve with cosmetic procedures?"

"I want to look perked up and fresh. But you can forget about surgery. I am afraid of going under the knife, and I do not want to look like one of those creatures I see all the time on the Upper East Side. You're not cutting me up and pulling my face back. No way!"

I assured her that's not what I do. Women and men come to me for non-invasive anti-aging procedures because they avidly hope to avoid cosmetic surgery. My use of fillers and Botox is very conservative. Barbara had tried both before, but the doctor had gone overboard and given her a hard, frozen look that she hated.

"Barbara, I promise you, I will keep you looking natural. When you walk out of here, no one will know you've had a cosmetic procedure. My approach is to simply make you look younger and more refreshed, as if you've just come back from the most incredible vacation of your life."

I could see she liked the notion. Even though I made it clear to her that it would take time, commitment, and money—one Thermage treatment alone can cost around $2,500, while a course of Botox and filler can add up to at least another $2,000—Barbara was more than ready to put in the work and investment if it meant turning back the clock on her terms.

First, I used Botox, sparingly, to smooth out her crow's feet. Then I injected some filler, Sculptra, into strategic spots underneath her cheekbones to smooth out the nasolabial folds—those marionette lines that run between the sides of the nose and mouth—and build some overall volume into her face. Over time, the filler would help her produce more collagen on her own, to thicken and tighten her skin.

On her next visit, I treated her neck and jawline with Thermage, a radio-frequency therapy that heats the deepest layer of the skin to stimulate collagen and tighten as it heals. I used the same treatment on her upper eyelids to open them up and eliminate some of the droop at the sides.

On her third visit, to keep her skin wrinkle-free and even out her skin tone, I started her on Fraxel, a laser therapy that's used over a course of multiple treatments. To help her maintain a smooth, glowing look, I also custom-blended prescription-strength compounds for Barbara to use at home, morning and night, to protect against environmental stresses during the day and to reverse the damage and rejuvenate the skin at night. They take only a few extra minutes a day to apply, and the long-term benefits will sustain her youthful appearance for years to come.

The results of this multipronged approach were subtle, just as I had promised, and the improvement was gradual. It takes 3 to 6 months to see final results with Thermage, but by then Barbara had turned back the clock by at least 5 years. Now, 7 years later, Barbara looks even better than she did after the initial round of treatments. She's been coming in twice a year for peels and maintenance shots of Botox and once every 2 years for Sculptra, and she sticks to her at-home skin care routine religiously. Her friends and family tell her she doesn't look a day over 45, and I know she will continue to look this good well into her next decade. She couldn't be happier.

"Thank God you didn't make me look like a freak," she exclaimed to me recently. "I didn't want to go through the rest of my life looking like I'm sitting in a wind tunnel. I feel like myself, only much, *much* better."

YOUR AGE, AND BEAUTIFUL

When I see pictures of Katharine Hepburn at any age, I think, "That's how a woman is supposed to age." She looks beautiful in her twenties, forties, sixties, and eighties. She was a stunning octogenarian. Sure, she had a few age spots and lines toward the end of her life, but so what? She took good care of her skin, and it showed all the way into her final years. Had she lived the majority of her life in this century, with access to all the age reversal technology we have today, she could have looked even lovelier for her years. And perfectly like herself.

The era of knock 'em out, stitch it up, or pull it back is over. Less is more. We're on the cutting edge of a kinder, gentler anti-aging revolution that's so much more elegant and natural than the current norm. An older face has so much more going on that makes it attractive. If a woman takes care of herself from an early age, she grows into her face beautifully. Her features tell a story about who she is.

Of course, everyone has a different aesthetic. When you're consulting with a dermatologist or a cosmetic surgeon, it often helps to bring in a photograph from a time when you felt you looked your best. Seek to restore the beauty that's already there.

GRADUAL REFINEMENT

We don't age overnight, and we should not expect to convincingly undo the damage with one quick fix. According to a recent study by the American Society for Dermatologic Surgery, about 89 percent of women said they would prefer a gradual effect that lasts 2 years over a dramatic change that lasts less than a year.[1] Patients are seeing much more natural and lasting results when they undergo a procedure like Sculptra, which slowly fills lines and folds through the stimulation of their own collagen and replicates their natural facial support platforms, or Thermage, which tightens skin over time. Lots of patients, however, aren't aware of these kinder options, and their doctors aren't informed enough to offer them.

A lot of science has gone into these solutions for the most gentle and natural age reversal. For every marker of aging, from pore size to skin elasticity, there is a specific technology or treatment that will address the problem. And it's not about having a specific procedure at a specific age. Everyone's skin ages differently. You could be 60 years old with the skin of a 40-year-old. Or, if you smoked and baked in the sun most of your life, you could be 40 with the skin of a 60-year-old. That is why the best approach is individualized and problem-specific.

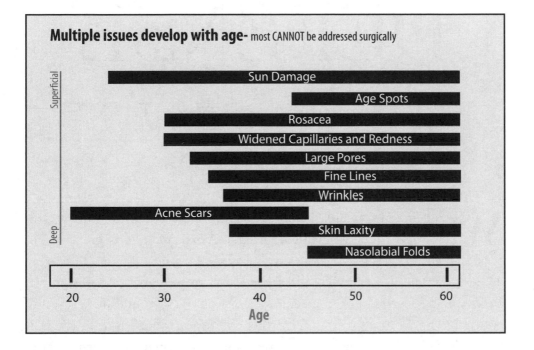

Multiple issues develop with age- most CANNOT be addressed surgically

With constant advances in technology, treatments such as lasers, radiofrequency, cell therapy, and advanced, collagen-stimulating fillers are better, safer, more comfortable, and far more powerful than anything that was available just a few short years ago.

I will talk about these and many more cutting-edge treatments in subsequent chapters. But in lockstep with these advances, patients and their doctors need to embrace a change in mind-set: Perfected and pulled is *out;* natural, healthy, and refreshed is *in.* The beauty to strive for is *you,* only better.

CHAPTER TWO

THE BEST DEFENSE

PROTECT NOW OR REGRET LATER

When I first met Cheryl, I couldn't believe she was only 30. She was an outdoorsy young woman who lived in Arizona and took great care of her body, but she was having issues with excessive pigmentation and freckling on her skin. She also had all the classic markers of the extrinsic aging caused by sun damage: wide pores, discoloration, fine lines around her eyes, and noticeable horizontal grooves across her forehead. I knew right away that Cheryl had been lax about sun protection. I was particularly concerned about a two-toned mole on the side of her nose. Fortunately, a biopsy revealed that it wasn't cancerous. But a melanoma would be in her very near future if she didn't change her ways immediately and do everything she could to protect her skin from UV rays and other environmental stresses. I read her the riot act. Fortunately, it wasn't too late for Cheryl. She came to me in the nick of time.

As a dermatologist, I see cases like Cheryl's every day, and not everyone is so lucky. It amazes me how so many of my patients are conscientious about their heart health, their diet, their blood pressure, and their general physical fitness yet do nothing to take care of their largest and most vital organ: their skin. The damage is particularly bad among my baby boomer patients. So much of the photoaging I see in my patients started when they were children or babies on the beach, slathered in baby oil by their well-meaning parents. Women in their fifties didn't know all that we do now about sun damage and skin cancer risks. Now they're paying the price.

HALF-COVERED

Even today, people make fatal mistakes in how they use sunblock, and they rely too heavily on products that don't do the whole job. No matter how scrupulous you think you are being, you are more than likely only partially protected: not even combating a third of the environmental stresses that can prematurely age your skin. And many of us have no idea how much damage we are exposing ourselves to just by going outside on a day-to-day basis. Just because you don't have a burn doesn't mean you haven't harmed yourself. You don't have to lie on a beach with a foil reflector or baste yourself with tanning oil to age your skin. It takes a lot less exposure to cause damage. Even when you are out running errands on a cloudy day, you are vulnerable; so to be safe, you should apply an SPF every day. It should be as automatic as brushing your teeth in the morning. Your skin is your body's largest organ. Why wouldn't you want to give it full protection?

Sun protection is also important for dark or African American skin. Just because the incidence of skin cancer is lower in black skin doesn't mean it can't happen. On the *Today* show recently, comedian Chuck Nice joked, "The sun doesn't know I'm black." He was sharing one of his favorite "things"—sunscreen with SPF 50—on the Kathie Lee and Hoda segment of the show. I wish all my patients were so enlightened. Yes, darker skin does have a little more built-in sun protection than white skin. But it can still burn, and when African Americans do get skin cancer, it's usually the more deadly kind.

Adam, my chief of operations, isn't always as diligent about protecting his skin as he should be, and a few years ago he had a face full of freckles. We corrected them with a light laser peel using the MedLite C6 laser—a tool designed for tattoo removal and treatment of excess pigment. The C6 delivers short, rapid, high-intensity pulses of light that target the melanin in your skin—even the spots you don't see on the skin's surface. Downtime is minimal, but as the skin heals, all the imperfections of the dermis are brought to the surface, which crusts a little before it peels off to reveal clearer skin. As Adam's face started to heal, a strange thing happened. A cluster of dark brown spots suddenly appeared on the left side of his face.

"Yuck! Dr. Sadick, what *is* this? How come the left side of my face has so much more pigment than the right side?"

"Well, Adam, the answer is a lot more simple than you might think. You do drive every day, don't you?"

"Sure, but I'm not outside in the sun."

"That's irrelevant. The sun's most damaging rays can burn right through your car window. Think about it. If you're sitting in the driver's seat on a regular basis, the left side of your face is going to get hit with the most UV exposure, assuming you aren't using sunscreen on your daily commute."

He wasn't. It had never occurred to him that he would need protection inside his car. But seeing what the sun was doing to his skin, and what he would have faced had he not treated his skin, was a good wake-up call. He was lucky one of those dark spots wasn't melanoma. Now Adam wears SPF every day.

The effects of the sun and the environment on our skin are insidious. And the damaging effects of free radicals—atoms or molecules in the atmosphere (pollution and sunlight) that can cause a chemical reaction on skin cells similar to the rusting effects of oxidizing agents on metal—as well as UVA and UVB rays can linger in our skin for hours after the sun goes down. In a car, beside a window, even when it's cloudy outside, you are still vulnerable; so when in doubt, apply that SPF. You won't regret it.

START NOW!

It is never too early or too late for prevention and protection. They are the biggest favors you can do for your skin and your overall health, whether

RISK FACTORS FOR SKIN CANCER

◆ Fair skin and hair; light-colored eyes; numerous moles; a personal or family history of skin cancer

◆ Major and repeated sunburn, especially before the age of 15

◆ Excessive artificial UVA tanning

◆ Immune suppression (from chemotherapy, infections, organ transplants—because transplant patients must take immune suppression drugs to treat HIV, lupus, and other conditions that compromise the immune system)

you are 20 or 60. Prevention can halt the onslaught of aging, and certain products can even help reverse damage. But skin protection must continue over the course of a lifetime. No exceptions. I don't care how young and beautiful you are, if you fail to protect your skin, even as a child, you'll see the damage in 5 to 10 years in the form of wrinkles, wide pores, rough patches, and even skin cancer. You could very well be putting your life in jeopardy. It's just not worth it. And if you neglect to protect your skin later in life, all that money you're investing in procedures and expensive skin creams will be wasted. Here are some particularly startling statistics regarding sun damage:

• One out of every five Americans—20 percent!—will get some form of skin cancer.

• Only half of Americans use the recommended dosage of sunscreen while exposing themselves to the sun.

• Nearly 30 million Americans use indoor tanning beds each year.

• UVA rays are the number one cause of skin aging.

• There has been a 300 percent increase in the incidence of melanoma skin cancer since 1994.[2]

I predict we're going to uncover more and more cases of skin cancer as our diagnostic tools improve. Instead of invasive and painful biopsies, doctors will soon be able to take quick digital and nonsurgical biopsies of your suspicious moles and accurately diagnose them on the spot. In 5 years, these devices could even be available at your local pharmacy, just like blood pressure machines. The disease will be easier to detect at an earlier stage, and we'll see more cases among the aging children of the 1960s, '70s, and '80s who did not know in their youth what we know about sun protection today.

AVOID THE AVOIDABLE

As a doctor, I am deeply upset to see such devastating effects from an entirely preventable condition. I have a 16-year-old daughter who is fair like me, with perfect porcelain skin, and she is never allowed out of the house without full sun protection. Your skin deserves the same loving care and concern. So here's what you can do about it, starting now:

First, we're going to take a look at the best protection you can buy. Not all sunscreens are created equal. An SPF is not enough. You need a broad-spectrum product—one that blocks not only the burning UVB rays, but also UVA rays—those insidious forces that can penetrate deep below the epidermis, the outermost layer of the skin, to the dermis, the inner layer of skin that contains blood vessels, glands, and hair follicles. UVB rays are harmful because they can burn your skin and cause skin cancer and other kinds of sunburn, and they operate between 10:00 a.m. and 4:00 p.m., particularly on sunny days. That's why most people think they need protection—to block the burn. But in many ways, UVA rays are worse. They go to work at all hours of the day, in sun, rain, or shine, and penetrate the protective layer of the epidermis, where they can hit blood vessels, nerves, and connective tissue. Damage, including carcinomas, deep wrinkles, excessive pigmentation, and even a weakened immune system, can show up years later. The danger of wearing a simple UVB sunblock is that you think you're more protected and may be more inclined to go out in the sun. But you're not safe at all.

Until recently, the popular wisdom was that there is no way to protect yourself against all of the sun's damaging rays. But now you can buy full-spectrum sunscreen with Helioplex. Neutrogena and La Roche-Posay make great products with this complex and similar formulations, which are available at most drugstores, and my clinical research staff also likes La Roche-Posay's Anthelios SX, Olay Complete SPF 30 Defense, and Clinique Sun. Just make sure when choosing a product that it has broad-spectrum UVA/UVB protection.

Sunscreen should also be photostable, meaning it can be stored for several weeks without losing its efficacy. And it should be non-irritating. Patients often give me the excuse that sunscreen is too harsh on their sensitive skin, or it blocks their pores and causes breakouts, but that's no longer the case with new formulations. If you can deal with their pastiness and opacity, use the sunblocks with zinc or titanium that don't allow any UV light to penetrate. Cosmetically, they have not been very elegant in the past, but soon there will be complete sunblocks on the market with ingredients that are so microscopically tiny, they are transparent on the skin. A good one available now is SkinCeuticals Physical UV Defense SPF 30.

Meanwhile, pay attention to the SPF numbers. A foundation with SPF 15 simply won't cut it. SPF 20 is sufficient for most people, but if you have lighter skin, or you live in the Tropics, you may need 30, 45, or 60. Apply it every day, even when it's cloudy, and at least every 3 or 4 hours if you are sweating or swimming. If you're bald, wear a hat. If you are lying on the beach, which is never a good idea, sit under an umbrella. That overbaked orange peel look is not in vogue anymore, not to mention extremely dangerous.

Even if you think you've been good about using sunscreen your whole life, chances are you weren't totally diligent about application. There are always areas we miss, either by accident or on purpose. Some people think it's okay to leave their legs exposed because they "already have a base there" and want a deeper tan. Others forget the tops of their ears or overlook their underarms. But there are new products on the market that integrate sunscreens so we can get that coverage despite ourselves. Wash-On by Aquea Scientific is a face and body wash that provides complete sunscreen protection simply by lathering up in the shower. Many brands of makeup, lipstick, and moisturizer now contain sunscreen, but on their own, they're not enough. You need that base coat of SPF on your face to greet the day.

And stay tuned. Within the next year, the FDA is going to require sunscreen manufacturers to rate the product's level of protection against UVA rays with one to four stars to let you know just how complete your protection will be.

WEAPONS UPGRADE

Even if you're using the best broad-spectrum sunscreen available, you're still not completely protected. A high-potency antioxidant is also essential for early prevention. Without it, you might as well be walking in a rainstorm without an umbrella. You need this powerful weapon in your arsenal.

An antioxidant should be applied first thing in the morning, before your moisturizer, to reinforce the protection of your sunblock, which goes on last. It often takes the form of a light cream or a serum, which contains finer formulations that allow the ingredients to soak in deep, past the epidermis. Think of it as that first of many lines of defense in your daily environmental shield.

An antioxidant acts like a scavenger, like a little Pac-Man, eating and neutralizing the damaging molecules that are in the air we breathe every day. Not only does the antioxidant help provide an extra weapon against the sun's rays, it protects against free radicals, which (to remind you) are particles in the atmosphere that can cause a harmful chemical reaction, called oxidation, on skin cells. Oxidation is basically the body's reaction to oxygen. So why is that bad? Paradoxically, oxygen provides life, but it also has a corrosive quality. Oxidation causes metal to rust, and it has a similar effect inside our bodies and on our skin. People throw around the term *free radicals* without fully understanding what they are, and as a result, the concept of protecting yourself against these molecules hasn't been taken seriously enough. But the danger

SUNSCREEN TIPS

◆ Avoid exposure between 10:00 a.m. and 4:00 p.m., when the sun's rays are strongest.

◆ Apply broad-spectrum sunscreen daily (UVB and UVA protection), preferably SPF 20 or higher, after your moisturizer and antioxidant or second to last if you wear makeup.

Here are some of the most effective sunscreen compounds:

- Avobenzone (Parsol 1789): A superior UVA blocker that is photodegradable (50 to 90 percent lost within an hour of UV exposure)
- Helioplex (avobenzone + oxybenzone + octocrylene = stabilized Parsol 1789)
- Ecamsule (Mexoryl SX): A photostable UVA + UVB blocker that is water-resistant and available in Anthelios SX

◆ Protect lips with a lip balm containing an SPF of at least 15.

◆ Use extra caution near water, snow, and sand, which intensify sun exposure by reflecting the sun's rays.

◆ Apply an ultrapotent antioxidant before your sunscreen to potentially augment its effect and offer further protection against free radical damage.

◆ Reapply sunscreen often (at least 1 ounce per application).

posed by free radicals is very real, and the cosmetics industry is finally catching up to that reality with a host of new and effective products.

RADICAL RECIPES

The most common antioxidant is vitamin C, but since this ingredient is unstable, it needs to be combined with others, particularly vitamin E and, to some extent, vitamin A. Together, these ingredients produce a synergistic effect that not only protects cells from free radical damage, but also helps skin rebuild its own collagen.

Other types of potent antioxidants are derived from various foods and plants, such as green tea, chocolate, red wine, lycopene (from tomatoes), licorice root, pomegranates, blueberries, and grape seed extract. Used in various combinations, the components can also help reduce inflammation and repair existing sun damage. The trendiest antioxidant ingredients these days are CoffeeBerry, an organic compound that uses the whole fruit of the coffee plant and is rich in polyphenols and resveratrol, a potent antioxidant derived from the grapevine. Other developments we are seeing in next-generation skin care are cocktails such as Biocell SOD (superoxide dismutase), which is a powerful combination of antioxidants. (More on all of these antioxidants in Chapter 6.)

Many of these ingredients are also good for your internal organs and can be ingested. I particularly like resveratrol, which is available in pill form and in topical formulations. I keep a bottle of supplement pills on my desk and take resveratrol twice a day. It fights skin cancer as well as prostate, breast, and lung cancers. Alkaloids, flavonoids, and carotenoids, which are in foods from coffee to tomatoes and carrots, are just a few of the other antioxidants that can be ingested for extra protection from the sun (I will also address internal solutions in Chapter 6). But if you want to have the most direct impact on your skin, topicals are the way to go.

Coenzyme Q10 (CoQ10) is another ingredient known for its antioxidant properties. Levels of this coenzyme occur naturally in the body and decline with age, but a topical version has been scientifically proven to improve uneven skin tone and wrinkles and penetrate the skin to reverse sun damage. Donell Super-Skin A+Q10, Mederma Scar Cream + SPF 30, DDF (Doctors Dermatologic Formula), Pangea Organics, Crème de Jour Multi-active by Colosé, and Avalon Organics are just a few of the brands that contain CoQ10.

Another interesting experimental drug that may have antioxidant properties similar to those of CoQ10 is idebenone. An organic compound of the quinone family, idebenone is starting to appear in topical creams, although it's mostly taken orally to treat neuromuscular disorders and diseases of the aging brain, like Alzheimer's. Idebenone can be found in the list of ingredients in Elizabeth Arden's Prevage, Radiance Revealing Complex, and Revitol Anti Wrinkle Complex. There's some debate over which antioxidants are more effective, but the molecules of idebenone are smaller than those of many other antioxidants and are therefore more readily absorbed by the skin. Idebenone may also be more effective at protecting cells against damage from reduced blood flow. However, more research is required to substantiate these claims. For now, the jury is still out on its efficacy in treating the signs of aging, topically or otherwise.

Look for products that contain some or all of the antioxidants I have mentioned here. In one of the prescription formulations I created for my patients, I include vitamins A, C, and E, green tea extract, and CoQ10. You can't have too many antioxidants working in your favor. I urge you to eyeball the ingredients yourself as you browse the shelves of Sephora or Duane Reade or Saks, but here are a few more products that contain some healthy antioxidant recipes, in no particular order: Caudalíe's Vinoperfect, Clinique Continuous Rescue, Christian Dior L'Or de Vie, La Crème (which I have tested in my research lab), Estée Lauder Re-Nutriv, and Lancôme Primordiale. Some of these are pricey, as many skin care products with the newest patented formulations and rare ingredients tend to be. But the beauty of antioxidants is that you have an extensive menu of options to choose from. Make a list of ingredients to look for and go to any cosmetics counter or your local drugstore to find something in your price range.

In a clinical study published in the *Journal of Cosmetic and Laser Therapy* in the summer of 2010, researchers found that antioxidants not only complement sunscreen for full protection, they can also work as a sunscreen themselves[3], staying active for several days after application. This by no means suggests that you should forgo sunscreen. You need both for optimal protection.

But this study documented particularly impressive results from an extract of the *Cassia alata* leaf, a potent antioxidant chock-full of flavonoids and polyphenols—two great warriors in the fight against free radicals. This miracle herb, also known as the candle bush plant, grows in tropical climates and is easily available from renewable botanical sources. The researchers chose this antioxidant for its stable properties and its strength. It has been claimed medicinally as a laxative and an antimicrobial and antifungal agent, as well as a treatment for ringworm, athlete's foot, ulcers, and skin infection. But as far as sun and environmental protection is concerned, antioxidants such as this one are protective because they stimulate cellular defense mechanisms for a prolonged period of time. Think of it as an extra, deeper layer of armor against environmental stresses.

Science is constantly coming up with newer, better, and more stable antioxidant compounds, whether they're derived from nature, synthetically, or in combination. Recent reports find that vitamin C, ferulic acid, and phloretin (found in the skin and flesh of apples) can help protect humans from photoaging. These compounds are also good at penetrating the skin barrier, which allows them to stay with you and keep you protected.

Beyond sunscreen and antioxidants, other new ingredients in this protection recipe are Sunspheres—hollow polymer spheres that boost the efficacy of sun protection through light refraction. These molecules are able to redirect the energy to be absorbed by the sunscreen and reduce the amount of UVA/UVB rays that actually reach the skin. Another is Uniprotect PT-3, which I have recently added to my own products because it has been shown to protect against protein damage, stimulate protein repair, and offer complementary UV protection.

As you can see, we have a modern-day menu of highly protective options that can help keep us healthy inside and out, and the efficacy of products available to consumers is improving year after year. Yet so many of my patients still allow their sun protection regimen to slide. As a physician, I get a knot in my stomach every time I have to make that dreadful phone call informing a patient that his or her biopsy tested positive for cancer. Melanoma is one of the worst forms of cancer because it can spread to other tissues and organs in a heartbeat if it's not detected early and treated aggressively. It's the deadliest of all skin diseases. Protecting your skin is not just about staying young and beautiful. It is about staying alive.

On this note, I urge you to go for annual skin cancer screenings, which are easy and painless and covered under most insurance plans. Early detection is key to avoiding the spread of skin cancer.

CHAPTER THREE

P.M.— REVERSE, RENEW, RESTORE

GIVE YOUR CELLS A WORKOUT WHILE YOU SLEEP

Now comes the second part of your skin care regimen—reversal and rejuvenation. While your morning routine should focus on protection, nighttime is all about repair and renewal, and that comes from boosting cell turnover and stimulating collagen. Once again, it's never too soon or too late to kick-start your cell activity. Start as early as your mid-twenties and ramp it up as you approach your thirties, forties, and fifties. The older and more sluggish our cells get, the more we may need stronger active ingredients and different mechanisms and delivery systems. But the principle is always the same: Do whatever you can to regenerate and stimulate your skin cells. Replenishing those that are constantly dying is key to maintaining and rebuilding a youthful appearance at any stage in life. The rate at which we replace them determines how well we age. When we are babies, our soft, plump skin turns over approximately every 14 days. As teenagers, our cells turn over every 21 to 28 days. As we age, cell renewal slows down to every 30 to 40 days. At 50-plus, cell turnover can slow to every 3 months. *But it doesn't have to be this way!*

One of my long-standing patients, Peggy, could be the poster girl for the New Natural. At 61, Peggy is a top executive at a major fashion house, so she is under constant pressure to look young and beautiful, and she pulls it off with grace. And unlike many of her peers in her industry, she has never once gone under the knife.

"I'm too scared," Peggy admits. "Not of the actual surgery, but of how unlike myself I might end up looking."

These words are refreshing to me. I see so many women past the age of 45 who are trying to look 25, and it's obvious they are trying too hard. Instead, Peggy looks like a woman in her late forties who takes extremely good care of herself. She's from the Midwest, but she reminds me of those beautiful French actresses who never allow age to get the better of them. Peggy has a few laugh lines around her sparkling eyes, but the rest of her skin is flawless. Her small wrinkles give her face character, and she is totally willing to keep them.

"A little line here and there is okay with me," she says. "My skin is not as tight as I'd like it to be, but the alternative is not attractive."

Her skin is remarkably firm for a woman her age. Nothing sags, and there are no deep folds or jowls. Her forehead is completely smooth, like porcelain, yet she can move her eyebrows up and down and show expression. There's an old English saying that a woman of a certain age must make a choice: "face or figure." But not in Peggy's case. She is slim and physically fit, and there's a youthful plumpness to her skin and fullness to her midcheek area. Her pores are invisible, and her skin positively glows.

DIVIDE AND CONQUER: A.M. AND P.M.

There's a multitude of skin care products out there, and figuring out how to use them may seem confusing at first. But don't despair. It's really not that complicated. Your daily skin care regimen should be based on one simple rule: Protect in the morning, reverse and rejuvenate at night.

◆ **A.M.**—Think about protection and prevention. The products you use should incorporate sunblocks, antioxidants, and moisturizing and detoxifying agents. You are building a barrier of protection for your skin before you go out and face the world. Protect that precious skin you've got.

◆ **P.M.**—Your pre-bedtime ritual is all about reversal. Think about putting your skin to work to repair the daytime damage while you sleep. Use products with retinoids, regenerative agents such as cell stimulators, peptides, and growth factors, and anti-inflammatory agents. (More on these in Chapter 5.)

Peggy has redefined what it means to look stunning for her decade. The young women who work for me stare at her in awe when she pays me a visit. They all want to know how to follow in her footsteps.

So what's her secret? Cell turnover.

Sure, Peggy does all the right things in the morning by applying sunscreen and antioxidants, but it's the lifelong nighttime routine she has been following since the age of 15 that has given her the added advantage in her fight against aging. Peggy is not genetically blessed with good skin. Her mother suffered from acne and other skin problems, but she made sure her daughter avoided her mistakes by teaching her to be scrupulous about skin care. Peggy was consistent about cleansing, moisturizing, and exfoliating. Never in her life has she gone to bed with her makeup on. As she got older, she upgraded to the new facial scrubs and high-quality moisturizers that became available. If a certain product was new and cutting-edge, she made it her business to research it and give it a try.

In her thirties, she was among the first wave of patients to go for micro-dermabrasion twice a year at the dermatologist's office. She also tried deep skin peels. Clearing the dead cells and debris from her skin's top layer allowed for better circulation and helped stimulate new cell growth below the surface. It also created a better canvas so that moisturizers and other topicals could penetrate deeper. At home, two or three times a week, she applied a retinoid to her skin to maintain consistent cell turnover (more on retinoids later in this chapter). She used a weekly face mask and performed mechanical exfoliation with a granular scrub, careful not to overdo it and irritate her skin.

At about age 35, Peggy started to notice deep creases running from the sides of her nostrils to the outer corners of her mouth—those dreaded naso-labial folds. She tried bovine collagen injections, a revolutionary procedure at the time, to plump up her skin. She had to have skin allergy patch tests to make sure the treatment was biocompatible. But over the long term, the early use of collagen—along with a series of autologous fat transfers (injecting her own fat extracted from other areas of her body), Sculptra fillers, and Ther-mage, a deep-heating treatment using radiofrequency energy—probably helped to stimulate cells beneath the skin's surface.

The quality of the skin care available to Peggy got better over the decades. She knew all the beauty and fashion editors of major women's magazines, and they tipped her off about the latest hot products. If a topical or treatment was claimed to be safe and had some solid scientific research behind it, she added it to her beauty routine.

"You should see my medicine cabinet," she jokes. "It's overflowing."

BEAUTY PIONEER

When beauty editors first started buzzing about the restorative benefits of copper peptides, Peggy was ready to try them. Peptides are fragments of the proteins that are the essential building blocks of skin tissue. Certain of these peptides bind well to copper, so scientists were able to develop a compound of peptides and copper atoms that were used medically to heal wounds and skin lesions as well as gastrointestinal ulcers. Dermatologists have used cop-per peptides for decades to help reduce scarring after various procedures like

ZAP IT!

You don't have to live with acne. Cutting-edge laser treatments, including at-home devices, can eliminate the problem and prevent long-term damage like scarring and dryness. This is critical. Patients prone to pimples tend to avoid treating their skin with age-preventing creams for fear of breakouts, even though many suffer from acne well into their thirties, forties, and even fifties.

Acne is a skin disease that affects more than 85 percent of teenagers. In many cases, acne diminishes with age, but I am seeing an increasing number of older patients with the condition. Acne can be treated by a number of over-the-counter remedies that contain drying agents such as salicylic acid or benzoyl peroxide. For more severe cases of acne, patients may opt for low-dose oral antibiotics, topical antibiotics, topical retinoids, phototherapy, or laser treatments. Heat and light delivery technology, which is available at the dermatologist's office or through at-home handheld devices, is also effective at reducing acne: speeding up the process of healing by shrinking the sebaceous glands.

Much simpler solutions include applying a warm washcloth to the area to stimulate the body's wound-healing response or a cold soy-milk compress to reduce inflammation.

Whatever you do, avoid excessive application of any topical acne product in the panic of trying to zap the zit. You don't want to dry out the skin and hurt the surrounding cells. You should continue to use a light moisturizer, and of course sunscreen, even when you suffer from breakouts.

And don't pick! You can't force the life cycle of an acne lesion. Trying to force it will only lengthen the healing process and possibly leave a permanent reminder in the form of an unsightly scar.

laser peels, and the skin care industry started to include these agents in their products a few years ago.

The compound works by synthesizing various components of the skin matrix and regulating the growth of certain types of cells. It's also a powerful anti-inflammatory, which aids the healing and renewal process. The jury is still out on how this ingredient works on wrinkles, but since wrinkles are essentially injured and degraded skin not dissimilar to wounds and scars, copper peptides could work in the same way, by promoting and stimulating the growth of regular collagen and reducing damage caused by the daily wear and tear on skin. Peggy certainly noticed some benefits. Her skin felt smoother and her pores were less visible. But she's since moved on to some even more cutting-edge products.

Today, Peggy's nighttime beauty routine consists of gentle cleansing, alternating between a soy-based cleanser and Christian Dior's Cleansing Water. She follows this with the new Capture Totale One Essential Skin Boosting Super Serum from Dior, which contains antioxidant ingredients like extract of the alpha longoza plant and a type of algae that either eliminate toxins or convert them into healthy proteins. Then, after laying the foundation, Peggy breaks out her Dior Capture Totale Serum, a creamy balm that helps boost the skin cells' metabolism, helping to create new cells more quickly, and firms the skin. She then applies eye cream, Dior's L'Or de Vie, and finishes with Capture Totale night cream, another cocktail of advanced ingredients that includes the longoza complex and fatty acids along with Centuline, a yeast derivative that prolongs the life span of cells, and calamansi, an extract from a type of citrus fruit that repairs cell damage and corrects pigmentation.

Peggy's whole nighttime ritual takes about 15 minutes. She massages each serum and lotion into her face in gentle upward motions, allowing a couple of minutes for each layer to sink in. It's not unusual for her husband to shout, "What are you doing in there? Come to bed!" But she never cuts it short. Peggy's morning ritual is similar, although it takes her only 10 minutes and involves different ingredients and creams after the cleansing process. It adds up to thousands of hours over a lifetime—and thousands of dollars in high-end skin care products. It's labor-intensive and time-consuming. But it's well worth it because she looks nothing like a woman in her seventh decade. Her skin quality is that of a well-preserved woman in her early forties, and she looks more beautiful and natural than anyone her age who has gone under the knife.

Consistency has been a key factor in Peggy's lifetime skin care regimen. Peggy has had access to the best and most expensive skin care ingredients that the beauty industry has to offer, but all those ingredients do little if you don't use them strategically and apply them daily. Peggy made the decision early in her life to make prevention, reversal, and renewal a priority, and before she became my patient, she knew instinctively that she needed to use whatever means she had at her disposal to promote cell turnover. I believe Peggy's commitment to nighttime renewal has played a larger role than the products themselves in making her the stunning 61-year-old she is today.

NEVER TOO EARLY

Early adoption is key. One of the biggest trends in cosmetic dermatology is the wave of young people seeking anti-aging treatments. My office sees a stream of patients under 30—often beauty-savvy fashion models—and it's not just for the odd pimple. They're getting Botox, laser resurfacing, micro-dermabrasion, injections of cell therapies . . . whatever it takes to keep their youthful looks and undo the damage of free radicals and the effects of smoking, alcohol, and sun damage on their skin.

You'd be surprised how much maintenance and prevention work goes into the flawless faces of models and actresses. Some of these women are models for beauty companies, and beauty is a highly competitive business that demands perfection: tiny pores and a blemish-free skin surface. Natural beauty takes work, and these girls know it.

The younger you start, the longer lasting the benefits. But whatever is true for my younger patients is *especially* true when you are older. The contrast in speed of cell turnover between your teens and your later decades is striking, but there are plenty of ways to get your cells back up to speed when you are past middle age. And unlike Peggy, my younger patients have access to a vast array of scientifically proven compounds that were unheard of when she was in her twenties and thirties. For these women, 60 could easily become the new 40 if they adopt Peggy's lifetime habits.

ESSENTIAL INGREDIENT

I'll talk at greater length in a later chapter about the more sophisticated new anti-aging formulas. But let's start with the gold standard of anti-aging ingredients. Retinol, the purest and most active form of vitamin A, has been

TOO MUCH ROSE

Ever notice yourself blushing, even when you're not embarrassed? Does a glass or two of wine at night leave you looking flushed the next morning? Does an afternoon out in the sun turn your face pink for days? Chances are you have rosacea, a widespread skin condition that affects about 16 million Americans, usually Caucasians (this is probably where the term *English rose* came from). Rosacea patients have flushing and redness on their faces, and as the condition worsens, they may also develop small pustules. The condition affects both sexes but seems to occur primarily in women ages 30 to 70. Those of German, Irish, and English descent are particularly prone to it. If you do have it, you are in good company. Famous rosacea sufferers include former president Bill Clinton, Princess Diana, W. C. Fields, and Rembrandt van Rijn, the 17th-century Dutch painter.

Unfortunately, there is no proven cause of rosacea, nor is there one ideal solution. Some say it's caused by inflammation. Others say it's a type of acne. New research conducted by the National Rosacea Society suggests that rosacea sufferers may have a higher number of the microscopic mites known as Demodex, which are normally found on the skin[4]. Stress, sun, alcohol, caffeine, extreme temperatures, and certain spicy foods can all be triggers, and it's a good idea to know what you can avoid to minimize the outbreaks.

It is important not to ignore rosacea, because it can get progressively worse. What starts out as a slight blushing around the cheeks that comes and goes can develop into inflammatory rosacea, complete with redness and itchy bumps that cover the entire face and even the chest area. Bloodshot eyes, spider veins, pimples, and a red bulbous nose are other symptoms of a flare-up. If left untreated, it could develop into vascular rosacea, a permanent condition that affects the blood vessels to the point where they become much more visible. The cheeks and nose swell, and the skin becomes ultrasensitive. Other unappealing symptoms are dandruff, oily skin, and enlarged pores.

around for years. Vitamin A can be broken down into thousands of smaller components, including retinoic acid, or tretinoin, the active ingredient in the Renova and Retin-A products. All of these are key components in helping skin cell turnover.

Retinol belongs to the family of chemical compounds known as retinoids and is one of the few substances used in skin care whose molecular structure is small enough to penetrate deep into the dermis for lasting potency.

Treatments for all stages of rosacea vary, and a dermatologist should be consulted. In the meantime, avoid irritating topical lotions and cleansers and use sunscreens with a minimum of SPF 20. Prescription treatments can include both topical and oral medications. A dermatologist may recommend a photorejuvenation treatment. Here are some options to consider:

◆ For stage 1, pre-rosacea, consider taking antibiotics, including tetracycline, metronidazole, doxycycline, azelaic acid, minocycline, anti-inflammatory sulfur topical creams, MetroGel, Finacea (also azelaic acid), and the newest anti-rosacea topical, PyratineXR, which claims to reduce redness quickly through the use of plant-derived growth factors. Use these topical gels consistently to prevent and control breakouts. A mild retinoid like Differin can improve the condition over time, although stronger retinoids such as Retin-A will only irritate the skin and worsen symptoms.

◆ For stage 2, mild rosacea, try a light peel. Glycolic, lactic, and salicylic acids, the chemicals used in these peels, work as anti-inflammatory agents and can minimize redness and bumps. Red light LEDs (light-emitting diodes) such as the Omnilux may also be helpful at this stage.

◆ For stage 3, permanent and diffuse redness, your best bet is intense pulsed light therapy or vascular lasers, which destroy the inflamed blood vessels. The heat is mild enough not to damage surrounding skin tissue. But it's not a permanent solution. There is no permanent solution. The redness could come back 6 months after treatment.

Rosacea can be difficult to treat, and while several regimens have proven effective, the key is to be patient. It can take up to 1 to 2 years to get the condition under control.

Retinoic acid also enables a form of communication between cells that helps them function properly and promotes a healthy pace of cell renewal. As we age, tired, misshapen cells that are more common in older skin don't communicate very well, and when they become sluggish, retinol wakes them up and gets them moving again.

Next to sun protection, retinol is the one product you should definitely have in your medicine cabinet. It has been scientifically proven to allow the skin to improve its overall integrity, stimulate new collagen, and thicken the dermis—that second, deeper layer under the epidermis where damage starts and renewal begins.

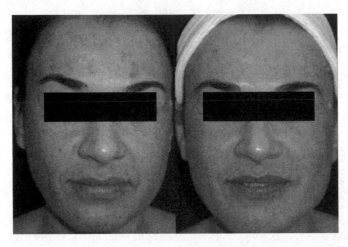

Daily application of Retinol over the course of 3 months softens nasolabial folds, smooths fine lines around the eyes, and improves overall skin texture, tone, and luminosity.

Retinol is time tested, and it works. After 6 months of consistent use, a group of 36 patients *over the age of 80* showed improvements in their skin quality that were visible to the naked eye, according to a 2007 study published in the *Archives of Dermatology*. The study tested an area of skin on each patient's arm following application of 0.4 percent retinol to the site three times a week for 6 months. Biopsies revealed more fibroblasts, elastin, and collagen—crucial building blocks for healthy skin cells.[5]

Consistent use of retinol-based topicals improves skin color, tone, and clarity by reducing pigment and helps slough off all those dead skin cells so that other restorative and firming products can penetrate deeper into the dermis. Removing dead skin cells also helps control adult acne by unclogging pores.

Retin-A is most specifically prescribed by dermatologists for its ability to improve the global appearance of fine lines, roughness, pigmentation, and sallow skin. But many other retinoid products are available over the counter that you can use to maintain the rate of cell turnover and keep skin looking

P.M.—REVERSE, RENEW, RESTORE 33

luminous. Look for these key ingredients: retinol, retinoic acid, retinaldehyde, and retinyl palmitate. Brands such as Renova, Tazorac, and Differin are all prescription products that contain retinoid and retinoid compounds that will keep skin clear and promote cell turnover, and safe and mild versions of retinol can also be found in many over-the-counter skin care products. In addition, alpha and beta hydroxy acids, derived from fruit, sugar, and plant sources, perform a similar cell renewal function. Beta hydroxy, also known as salicylic acid, is a useful alternative for people who are prone to acne because it promotes the shedding of skin cells. It also clears skin and helps reduce excessive pigmentation—the overproduction of melanin in the skin that causes liver spots, freckles, discoloration, and uneven skin tone—another issue that we tend to overlook until it becomes all too obvious.

EASY DOES IT

You may experience some sensitivity and redness when you use a retinoid. Many of my patients do, and in those cases I tell them to go for a lower concentration of the retinol derivative (the FDA allows up to 1 percent in over-the-counter brands). A gentler formulation is better than nothing at all. Anti-inflammatory ingredients used in combination with retinols can also help minimize the irritation and build the skin's tolerance to some of the stronger retinoid formulas. You can also minimize irritation by applying a moisturizer over the retinol.

If you don't want to have to go to your dermatologist for a prescription-strength retinoid, here's a list of retinol products currently available at the skin care counter. I am putting them in approximate order of strength, so that you can graduate to stronger formulas over time:

• Afirm 1X through 3X by Afirm—This product comes in three strengths, 0.15 percent for beginners, 0.30 percent for those with less sensitive skin, and 0.60 percent for those who have built up a tolerance and want more dramatic results

- Retinol Cream 15 by BioMedic

- Reversal by Sadick Dermatology Group

- Retinol Complex by SkinMedica

- Retinol Cream 60 by BioMedic

- Factor A Lotion by Jan Marini Skin Research

- Skin Perfecting Lotion by Murad

- Retinol Smoothing Serum 2X by Replenix

- High-Potency Serum by Cellex-C

- Topix Replenix Retinol Plus Smoothing Serum 10X—With green tea to reduce inflammation and sun sensitivity

- Peter Thomas Roth Retinol Fusion P.M.—Also with vitamins C and E

- SkinMedica Retinol Complex—With retinol, retinyl acetate, and retinyl palmitate and vitamin E

- PCA Skin Retinol Renewal Phaze 26

- RoC Retinol Correxion Deep Wrinkle Serum—Also with magnesium, zinc, and copper

- Retinol 1.0 Maximum Strength Refining Night Cream by SkinCeuticals— The most potent retinol product available without a prescription

Do not use these products daily, particularly the stronger formulations. Alternate them with other formulations twice a week to give your skin a rest, and if you experience sensitivity, try soaking gauze in some soy milk or regular milk and applying the compress to the affected area to soothe any irritation. If you have a fair complexion or sensitive skin, consider using soy-milk compresses. It really calms down the skin. And don't neglect areas off the face. Skin care shouldn't stop at the jawline. Use retinoids regularly on your neck, chest, and even your hands, and you'll stave off the signs of aging in those key areas as well.

I also recommend skin peels for my patients to boost cell turnover. They help promote circulation and create a more luminous surface. Plus, they scrub away those free radicals that can slow down cell production and make the skin appear more ashen and dull.

BE GENTLE

There are many different ways to promote cell turnover in addition to retinoids, but the more widely available skin care products tend to emphasize the mechanical turnover of cells through facial scrubs. A glycolic face wash is a nice, gentle way of getting rid of the gunk, but abrasive face washes can be tricky. St. Ives Apricot Scrub is a fine product, but don't overdo it because it doesn't work on the skin's deeper layers, and overuse of abrasion can lead to inflammation and redness. When it comes to at-home exfoliation and cleansing, less is more. If your skin feels particularly sluggish and dull, microdermabrasion or any kind of peel—laser or chemical—is a more effective method of skin cell turnover.

Remember, though: Products that promote cell turnover should be used at night, so your skin can recover while you are sleeping. If your skin is sensitive, your dermatologist can offer the most gentle methods. You don't want too much inflammation, but a little can be a good thing because it keeps the blood flowing and oxygenates the cells.

Whatever you do, make some sort of nighttime reversal regimen a lifetime habit. Consistency is key. The payoff will be obvious when you've reached your seventh decade looking as gorgeous and youthful as Peggy.

CHAPTER FOUR

TAKE IT HOME

BE YOUR OWN BEST DERMATOLOGIST

I hadn't seen Rebecca in about 2 years. She used to be a regular visitor to my practice because she suffered from chronic adult acne. Rebecca was 38 when she had her first big flare-up thanks to stress and hormone fluctuations after her first child was born. We got it under control with lasers and topicals, and every few months Rebecca would come back to see me—a visit that usually coincided with some other exacerbating stress factor in her life.

But after her last visit, she bought a small blue light LED (light-emitting diode) device designed specifically for treating acne at home. Like the professional medical device we use in my offices to treat acne, the handheld gadget uses heat and light to kill acne bacteria and heal inflamed, clogged pores. Holding it for 20 minutes every day over the areas of her face most prone to outbreaks was effective enough to keep her out of my office for a surprisingly long time. When she did come to see me again, a big promotion, more responsibilities, and the added stress of looking after an energetic toddler were wreaking havoc on her skin, and it was more than she could handle on her own. She needed a fast fix before an important meeting in 2 days, so I treated her with cortisone injections and a prescription-strength acne-clearing product we have developed in our office. Apart from that one area of her face that was affected, Rebecca's skin looked pretty good. Thanks to her high-tech at-home regimen, those severe and persistent acne outbreaks appeared to be a thing of the past.

These days, the newest technology isn't accessible only in a doctor's office. Besides keeping a stash of skin care products for morning protection and evening reversal (sunblocks, moisturizers, toners, retinoids, exfoliators, and antioxidants), those truly diligent about slowing down the clock can invest in moderately priced laser devices for use at home. They don't necessarily replace what a dermatologist can do for you, but for certain skin issues they can serve as a great adjunct to your beauty regimen, augmenting and prolonging whatever professional treatments you may receive.

Years ago, our practice was among the first to develop lasers and light sources for hair removal in a professional setting, and these devices proved to be powerful and highly effective. Now we have home hair removal systems that work like milder versions of the professional ones. On the skin care side, lower levels of light, heat, and radiofrequency treatments currently offered by dermatologists for stimulating collagen, tightening skin, and improving acne are starting to appear on the shelves of beauty retailers such as Sephora. They are relatively small investments that have the potential to offer substantial benefits over the course of a lifetime if you are persistent. Since they are much less powerful than professional technologies, consistent use is very important. If you are not willing to spend an extra 10 or 20 minutes a day, it may be better to save that $300 or so and put the cash toward your next visit to the dermatologist.

That said, second and third generations of home skin care technology could soon produce professional results. The menu of options is rapidly growing, with major beauty companies like L'Oréal, Johnson & Johnson, and Procter & Gamble scrambling to improve the technology and come up with more affordable gadgets that use everything from microcurrents to LEDs. The LED handhelds have tiny bulbs that operate at specific wavelengths depending on the skin issue you are trying to treat. Blue light zaps acne-causing bacteria, and red light targets wrinkles by stimulating collagen and reducing inflammation. It takes a committed regimen of 20 minutes a day for some devices, but results for acne treatment and hair removal are almost as good as what you can get from a doctor's visit, and the regimen costs less if you use the device often enough to pay for itself.

This is one of my shortest chapters because there aren't many at-home devices I consider effective enough to warrant much ink here. And for the handful I do like, there are many more ridiculous money wasters out there that make false claims. You know the ones I'm talking about. You see them on infomercials all the time: the Face Mask, which supposedly adds resistance to ordinary facial movements and thereby helps you strengthen facial muscles. There are several variations that make an exaggerated connection between facial muscle growth and skin laxity and wrinkles. You could go around all day wearing this thing, looking like Freddy Krueger, and still see no effect. The Neckline Slimmer is equally absurd, designed for you to press your chin onto its top while it pumps up and down, like an aerobic workout that helps you shed neck fat and tighten slack jowls. You might get a stiff neck and a headache for your troubles, but an Audrey Hepburn neckline isn't going to happen. Sorry.

If you would like to look like a character from *Star Trek,* you could also try Safetox. Proponents of this device—a blue plastic headband that looks like a space age fashion statement—claim it's an alternative to Botox without the pain. Electric impulses generated through an adhesive patch in the middle of the headband supposedly target the forehead muscles and relax them to reduce wrinkles. While you may get some temporary results, wearing this thing twice a day for 5 minutes over several weeks seems like a lot of trouble to go to when a few tiny pricks of a needle will produce much more dramatic results. Save your $488. Instead, consider investing in the Freeze 24-7 pocket-sized gadget for around $65. It delivers a metered dose of salve that contains numbing ingredients to temporarily freeze facial muscles and reduce wrinkles.

Its claims may also be a bit exaggerated, but at least you won't be shelling out too much cash!

Let me save you the trouble and give you a quick rundown of the newest beauty gadgets that might actually do something for your skin. These devices aren't all equally effective, but a few may be worth the investment.

HAIR REMOVAL

There are several new devices on the market that do a pretty good job of getting rid of unwanted hair. Some are more powerful than others, but the main difference is price, which varies depending on retailer, local taxes, and other regional factors:

• The Silk'n SensEpil—A broad-spectrum light source similar to an IPL (intense pulsed light) with a wavelength that ranges from 600 to 1,100 nanometers. It's about the size of a small travel hair dryer, with a light source at one end that emits a pulsed light. You run the device along the skin and click the pulse button on the handheld device, which flashes on the 2- by 3-centimeter area to be treated. The light comes with a cartridge, which usually lasts long enough to treat the whole body but costs about $55 to replace. It stores in a base unit the size of a facial tissue box, which has a panel that allows you to control the strength settings. The control panel also indicates when skin is too dark to be treated without burning. It's not recommended for use on the face and can be painful on the bikini area. The device has been FDA approved and costs about $575.

• Tria—Using diode laser technology, it has an 810-nanometer wavelength, one of the stronger systems that may also work on darker skin. It covers a 1- by 1-centimeter area, so it's good for targeted hair removal, but it may take longer to cover larger areas like the legs. The cordless device is more compact than the Silk'n and looks a little like a children's toy ray gun. It works in much the same way: When the device is placed on your skin, it will beep. Keep holding it there, making sure to maintain complete contact with the skin. It will beep again, letting you know that the section is completed.

SEASONAL SKIN

Whenever the seasons change, I get bombarded with questions surrounding what kind of impact the harsh weather has on the skin. While basic principles of good skin care never change, there are a few adjustments you may want to make depending on what climate you are in.

Many people ask if colder temperatures have medicinal or anti-aging benefits, but to date there are none known. In fact, winter is probably the toughest on skin, because the combination of dry air and extreme temperatures can cause dryness and irritation. Exposing your skin to freezing, windy winter weather can promote and contribute to aging. So how should you protect your skin during the winter months? I've always recommended that patients use a thicker, richer moisturizer than they would use during spring or summer to create a barrier against the elements. I also suggest that patients use moisturizers indoors during the winter months because heated rooms can cause skin to become dry and dehydrated. Using a humidifier is also a good idea. With that said, it's important to avoid both extremely hot and extremely cold temperatures because of their negative impact on skin.

When winter is in full swing, with temperatures hovering below freezing, many people experience dry, irritated, cracked, and chapped skin through their exposure to the extremes of outdoor and indoor temperatures. Winter can be especially challenging for patients with eczema, a common condition where the patient experiences skin dryness and recurring skin rashes.

The best way to prevent problematic winter skin is to keep it fully moisturized. The first and simplest step is to use a humidifier indoors. The additional moisture can eliminate or minimize a dry nose, prevent dry, itchy, or cracked skin, and help some avoid allergy and asthma problems. Most patients notice a difference in the severity of their dry skin immediately after the humidifier is in place.

If you hear a buzz instead of a beep, it means the laser treatment wasn't completed and you have to redo it. Work your way through the area, moving horizontally and overlapping the area you just treated by about a quarter inch. Do the same vertically to ensure that you don't miss any spots. The only inconvenience with the Tria is that it needs to be recharged every half hour. If you are treating a large area, you will have to interrupt the process to recharge and remember where you left off. The Tria is FDA approved and costs about $495.

The second step to reducing the symptoms of winter skin is to use a moisturizer with higher oil content. These moisturizers form a layer of protection that literally locks in moisture. Ointments are another good choice. An ointment is basically a water-and-oil emulsion that can contain up to 80 percent oil. You can also use any products on the market for "extra" dry skin. While these do not contain as much oil as ointment, they do have a higher oil content than traditional moisturizers, and this will definitely help protect and condition skin while reducing itchiness and redness. The greatest way to moisturize skin in winter months is to apply a moisturizer or ointment immediately after showering so you can lock in the moisture. Be sure to use warm (not hot) water for your showers. A hot, steamy shower or bath may feel great on a cold day, but it can actually make your skin feel worse. Opt for warm showers, and for best results pat your skin dry and immediately (and generously) apply a highly moisturizing lotion or ointment. This will help improve your skin and prevent it from drying out. Other helpful tips include dressing in layers to prevent the skin from becoming too cold (outdoors) or too overheated (indoors). Sweaty, moist skin combined with extreme temperatures can cause further irritation.

And don't think winter weather means you can skimp on sunscreen! Continue to use a broad-spectrum sunblock with an SPF of at least 20 every day. Whether you are skiing with your family or on the beach enjoying the sunshine, do not forget that the strongest sun exposure occurs between the hours of noon and 4:00 p.m. These are the times you should minimize your sun exposure. If you get sunburned, red light LED sources available from your dermatologist can accelerate healing, reduce redness, and decrease the potential for permanent damage in the form of discoloration or wrinkles.

Do whatever you can to protect your skin from the season's harshest elements.

• Epila SI 808 Laser—Uses a laser diode with an 808-nanometer wavelength and, like the other devices, uses a broad spectrum of light wavelengths. Its sleek design resembles a man's electric shaver. Users are instructed to shave the area first, then apply a cold damp towel to the area to be treated, to keep the skin's temperature low. Adjust the setting, starting at a lower strength, until you get a feel for how your skin will react. Place the touch bar of the Epila unit as close as possible to the area you wish to treat and push the laser button. As with the Tria, you should hear a beep when the laser is activated. Move the Epila unit in a slight circular motion as you activate the laser and not directly at the hair follicle. This allows the laser to penetrate beneath the skin and destroy the hair follicle at the root rather than at the point where the hair emerges through the skin. Use the system for no longer than 30 minutes at a time, then take a break to soothe your skin with the cool towel before resuming treatment. Always stop if you feel too uncomfortable or if you feel a burning sensation on your skin. Overall, Epila offers coverage similar to Tria's, but unlike the other devices, it has not yet been FDA approved and consumer reviews are mixed. Epila costs about $250.

All of these devices employ lower energies than those available in the doctor's office, so they take longer per procedure, and it will take many more treatments to achieve the results you could get more quickly in a professional setting. However, many are FDA approved and when used for longer periods of time (8 to 12 weeks) have produced decent (up to 60 percent) long-term hair removal in clinical studies. Results are almost comparable to what dermatologists are able to achieve in office settings. Plus, numerous published scientific studies have confirmed the safety and efficacy of these at-home technologies. For the consumer's sake, I am glad to see there is growing competition in the marketplace and that these beauty solutions are more accessible to everyone.

CELLULITE TREATMENT

I mention at-home cellulite devices only as a warning not to get lured by the hype of any that claim to improve the appearance of cottage cheese thighs. In my office, we have every kind of state-of-the-art professional body-contouring machine that's out there, and even I cannot promise complete cellulite resolution to my patients. The home market is full of cellulite "solutions" that are not backed by science and have proven to be largely ineffective. Here's one highly advertised device that came out in 2005:

• Wellbox Lipomassage LPG Machine—Combines suction and massage to break up the cellulite and claims to be quite the multitasker, not only taking care of orange peel thighs, but tightening sagging skin on the face, softening wrinkles, and relieving body aches and pains. Wow! That's quite a machine. But its many talents don't come cheap. The device, which requires a training video to understand how to use all five of its settings, retails for about $1,500. At most, you'll see a slight improvement in the areas of your body affected by cellulite because of the swelling and tightening effect induced by all that rolling and suction. But it won't last much more than a couple of hours. Skip it!

CLEANSING

At-home devices for exfoliation and cleansing have been around for a few years. Sloughing off dead skin cells is a good mechanical way to promote cell turnover, which is a necessary part of your skin maintenance regimen. For an extra boost, it's sometimes helpful to visit a dermatologist or a skin spa for microdermabrasion treatments to clear the skin's surface and make way for new cell growth. But nowadays, you can get near salon quality with some new devices on the market. Try:

• Clarisonic Mia Sonic Skin Brush—A compact cordless handheld device with an easy-to-grip handle and a brush about 2 inches across that oscillates more than 300 times a second to shake off those dead cells and smooth the skin's surface, creating a better canvas for all those cutting-edge cosmeceutical ingredients to sink deeper into the dermis. At about $150, it gets the job done, which is more than I can say about a lot of these gadgets.

HAIR GROWTH

There are also special brush devices that claim to stimulate hair growth, and they do have a minimal effect on some patients. Very minimal. If you are suffering from severe hair loss, you would be better off reviewing the complete range of treatments detailed in Chapter 14, but if you want to experiment at home with red light therapy before you take it a step further, here's one gadget you can try:

• HairMax Laser Comb—Works by delivering heat to the hair follicles and improving blood flow to the scalp. It looks like a cross between a small cordless phone and a bulky hairbrush, with a set of comb teeth on either side of the laser light. The treatment, which requires 15 minutes three times a week, may also help reduce inflammation on the scalp to prevent further hair loss. It costs about $495, so it's not cheap. As a hair loss expert, I humbly suggest you seek out the best professional treatment at the earliest signs of hair loss for the best results.

ACNE TREATMENT

As we saw in the case of Rebecca, at-home blue light devices are pretty effective at keeping certain kinds of acne outbreaks under control. They help reduce acne-forming bacteria, decrease inflammation on the skin, and temporarily shrink sebaceous glands. Ongoing FDA and published studies highlight the efficacy of at-home acne treatments used in combination with topical acne antibiotics, benzoyl peroxide, retinoic acid derivatives, and in some cases oral antibiotics. Most are small enough to slip into the palm of your hand, and some are no bigger than a lipstick case for on-the-go use. They work simply by applying directly to the pimple, zapping the bacteria with a small heat sensation or pinprick. Here are a few handheld gadgets that have been proven effective:

• Zeno Mini Acne Clearing Device—Delivers heat for about 2 minutes to shorten the pimple's life span and stop it from getting worse. The heat shock response in the skin causes the acne bacteria to self-destruct. Note that it may burn sensitive skin. The technology works well if you have an occasional pimple or two, but it may not be as effective on severe outbreaks. At around $89, it's not a bad deal considering a single cortisone shot can cost about $100 at the dermatologist's office.

• ThermaClear—Also uses heat elements but lays claim to more power in controlled pulses. The manufacturer also says it takes a shorter time to zap the pimple than its rival the Zeno, but both pocket-sized devices work equally well if you catch the pimple early enough. It costs about $150.

• Tanda Clear Acne Light Therapy—Uses blue light LEDs to deliver clinical levels of light. The handheld gadget is FDA approved and uses 414-nanometer wavelengths to treat existing blemishes and prevent future outbreaks. It may not be a complete cure, but it certainly helped keep Rebecca's acne under control. At about $350, it's also one of the more expensive of the zit zappers.

• Claro—Uses IPL technology, combining both heat and light, and is also FDA approved. It claims a 94 percent clearance rate for acne. This statistic may be a little optimistic, but as with these other devices, the few studies out there suggest it is also effective on moderate acne. Price tag: about $250.

While these at-home gadgets have proven successful in some cases, let me be clear. If you have severe or cystic acne lesions, they probably aren't going to give you what you need. They can work well in between doctor's visits and may help reduce the severity of outbreaks. But what pleases me about this proliferation of new devices is that patients are being introduced to the possibilities of technology. Patients may use them, find they work to some degree, and choose to go to a dermatologist for stronger versions of the same treatments. I see this at-home technology not as competition for my business, but as a complement to it.

FACIAL REJUVENATION

I am less impressed, on the other hand, with some of the claims device manufacturers make about their anti-aging capabilities. We've tested dozens of these machines at our research lab, and our assessments range from "worthless" to "minimally effective." I've decided to include a couple of the more dubious devices in our list simply because they are so prevalent in the marketplace and I don't want you to get seduced by the manufacturers' slick marketing claims. Bear in mind that the power output of these machines is a fraction of what you would get in the doctor's office. Even in clinical settings, patients may require multiple treatments from the most powerful lasers and radiofrequency devices, so you can imagine how much time and effort it takes to use at-home lasers to get a fraction of the rejuvenating and tightening effects of professional technology. Some of the following gadgets could be a nice bridge between doctor visits, but they are all very low-level technologies, and most have limited clinical research to back them up:

• NuFACE—The manufacturer describes this device as a "non-invasive face-lift with immediate results." You probably see it everywhere. NuFACE is a favorite on home shopping channels and in online catalogs, based on the principle that electronic impulses can tighten and contract the muscles of the face, thus improving circulation and tightening sagging skin. It has two probes that you run over your face and neck for 5 minutes after applying a conductor gel. Claimed benefits include improved pigmentation, reduced acne, shrinking of pores, elimination of fine lines and wrinkles, reduction of scars and pockmarks, and improvement of skin conditions like rosacea and eczema. Don't be fooled by the slick marketing. It's sheer nonsense. If NuFACE actually fulfilled its promise, we dermatologists would all be out of business. If you don't believe me, by all means take advantage of the money-back guarantee NuFACE's marketers offer through TV home shopping shows. You'll probably find that there is some slight (albeit very temporary) benefit from improved circulation. The buzzy feeling of the probe may even trick you into thinking the device is really doing something deep below the skin's surface. But after a while, you'll realize your face looks exactly the same. Be sure to send it back within the 30-day limit so you don't waste your money. Price tag: about $325.

• ilift—Here's another gadget that may sound as though it's based on science but is in fact useless. Made by a company called Laser.com out of Italy, the device looks more like a cell phone than a beauty gadget. The makers of this machine claim it uses negative and positive ions, microdermal massage (whatever that means), infrared rays, and, for an extra $75, a laser-lift serum to prevent and soften wrinkles, increase skin elasticity, and reduce facial muscle tension. In short, it supposedly does everything! This is one of those products that are hyped with a cocktail of buzzwords that sound good but have no basis in real science. Save your money. Price tag: about $395.

• Dual Ultrasound and Ion Therapy Sonic—Similar in claims to the ilift, this device purports to use ultrasound and ions to lift, tighten, and generally improve the texture of the skin. It has no effect. Price tag: about $325.

• ANSR—This blue and red light laser device is designed to treat acne (with the blue LED) and rejuvenate skin (with the red setting). The principles are fairly sound and based on in-office treatments, but the ANSR contains only a few LED bulbs and delivers a small fraction of the energy administered by office machines. It may be effective for treating one or two pimples at a time, but even that is doubtful. Price tag: about $130.

• The Baby Quasar Photorejuvenation Device—Another machine based on the principles of red light therapy. But again, it's not powerful enough to have an effect, so at $450 you would be wasting even more of your money. Likewise for LightStim ($349).

• Tanda Regenerate Right Light Therapy—You may have more luck with this LED system. The device uses 660-nanometer wavelengths of red light, which makes it a little more powerful than most of the other at-home red light gadgets on the market. The red light helps to promote the skin's natural healing process and stimulate the production of collagen. There's also a blue light head for the Tanda that works pretty well on acne. Used alone, the Tanda red light device will produce a minimal effect over time, but it may help maximize the benefits of clinical treatments. It could also give your skin care product an extra boost by helping the active ingredients sink deeper into the dermis. Be prepared to spend some quality time under this wand, however. The manufacturer recommends 18 minutes every day for the first month and two or three times a week after that. And it retails for around $395, so it's not cheap.

For the most part, these anti-aging devices are not as powerful as the machines you will find at the dermatologist's office, and neither are the results. The ANSR is a great example. Yes, it is based on red and blue LEDs, but just because it offers the same type of technology does not mean the energy, treatment protocol, and treatment time are the same. If you spend 20 minutes in my office under the full-face Omnilux LED red and blue light, you won't need to consider waving an ANSR gadget over your face.

For now, the best at-home technology focuses on acne and hair removal, but there is no question that at-home anti-aging is the direction of the future. Think of it like the early cell phone technology. The first phones were the size of shoeboxes with crackling reception, and today we can watch movies and surf the Internet on our phones. When it comes to at-home beauty technology, we're a little past the prehistoric cell phone stage, but we still have a long way to go. And we'll get there. In a few years' time, you may be able to do for yourself what you pay thousands of dollars for at the dermatologist's office. The momentum of progress is building and it can't be stopped, so keep your eyes and ears open. Meanwhile, be critical when you are browsing through a Brookstone catalog or watching the Home Shopping Network for products.

PART II

MAINTAIN

(Ages 30 to 80 . . .)

CHAPTER FIVE

LOTIONS AND POTIONS

WHAT STEM CELLS CAN DO FOR YOU

The last 2 years have seen incredible advances in cosmeceuticals, or cosmetic products with biologically active ingredients purporting to have medical or pharmaceutical benefits. These compounds have been proven especially effective at filling out fine lines, tightening pores, and evening out skin tone. Some can even thicken and plump the outer layer of the skin for a more youthful appearance. But if you don't believe me, I commend you for your cynicism. There's a lot of clutter out there, and it takes a degree in biochemistry to sort out the credible claims from the false advertising.

Let me take this moment to offer full disclosure. I am paid to work as a medical consultant with several brands, including Christian Dior and Avon. My practice also has its own prescription-strength products and is working on a new consumer anti-aging line. That means my clinical research company

BUYER BEWARE

The Seven Most Common Cosmeceutical Myths

While the cosmeceuticals I recommend in this book have proven track records for safety and efficacy, it's always wise to exercise caution when purchasing products not directly prescribed by your dermatologist. Here are some of the more common false assumptions about cosmeceuticals to bear in mind on your next trip to the cosmetics counter:

◆ Cosmeceuticals and cosmetics are regulated by the FDA as drugs.

◆ Cosmeceutical claims/labels/advertising are substantiated and approved before the product reaches the market.

◆ Cosmetic ingredients undergo premarket testing by the FDA for safety.

◆ Cosmetic ingredients undergo premarket testing by the FDA for efficacy.

◆ "Natural" ingredients are safer than synthetic.

◆ "Cruelty-free" means no animal testing.

◆ Hypoallergenic means something. (Not really. It is mostly an advertising term.)

tests these (and other) products, recommends ways to improve them, and suggests protocols. It does not mean I profit directly from their sales. Whenever I work with a company, or even on my own products, I always include a clause in my contract that states that I will only endorse products with good scientific research and the highest standards of safety and efficacy. When I recommend a product in these next pages, I will at all times try to include a list of comparable brands or ingredients that have been clinically tested by Sadick Research Group or another dermatology lab. If I don't believe something works, I will say so.

Involving dermatologists in the development of these commercial products is great for the consumer, because it raises the bar for efficacy. Certain bioactive ingredients used in cosmeceuticals do indeed have an effect beyond the traditional moisturizer. But let's be clear: *Cosmeceutical* remains a marketing term not recognized by the FDA. Developers have no legal obligation to prove that the products actually live up to their claims. And cosmeceuticals are not required to undergo the same rigorous testing and quality control as pharmaceuticals, which are more potent and would be prescribed by a physician.

Depending on your particular skin issue, cosmeceuticals may not be an adequate substitute for compounds developed and prescribed specifically for you by your dermatologist. They do not always treat medical conditions of the skin like psoriasis or eczema as effectively as a prescription medication, so if you are using them for those problems, have your doctor verify that they don't interact adversely with what is being prescribed for you. You can roughly gauge an ingredient's potency by where and how it appears on the product label. If it's listed at the top, you'll know it's one of the product's primary ingredients. Generally speaking, the percentage of active ingredients in cosmeceuticals is much lower than that in prescribed agents, and most cosmeceuticals cannot make dramatic claims. However, that does not mean they are not effective for most people looking to improve the overall texture and quality of their skin. These products are getting better and better every year.

Beauty and skin care companies like Christian Dior, Procter & Gamble, and Johnson & Johnson are pouring millions of research dollars into double-blind studies (clinical trials in which neither the participating individuals nor the study staff know who is receiving the experimental drug and who is receiving a placebo, to prevent bias). They know it's worth making the investment as the population ages and demands better products. A growing number of skin creams and serums now on drugstore and department store shelves have come straight out of the science labs. Dior, Neutrogena, Oil of Olay, and Avon all have cosmeceutical product lines with ingredients that have been researched, proven, and written up in peer-reviewed periodicals like the *Journal of Drugs in Dermatology,* a highly respected publication that now has to produce frequent supplementary issues to keep up with the fast pace of research and development in this field. There are other, smaller brands at Sephora or even your local drugstore that are safe and effective. You just need to know which components to look for.

The price range of these products is vast. A 1-ounce jar of Crème de la Mer costs about $130 at Saks and half an ounce of Dior's L'Or de Vie L'Extrait retails for around $261 because both are made with ingredients that are difficult to procure, harvest, or extract. Small quantities of these ingredients are formulated with other extremely high-quality extracts or compounds to create a highly concentrated and bioactive product. You will get much more noticeable results from one of these products than from a lotion or cream you can buy for $9 at Walgreens. Are they absolutely necessary to your skin care regimen? No. But if you can afford them, rest assured you are not throwing your money away. They are worth the higher price.

Unlike many beauty and skin care products of the past whose claims were either exaggerated or unfounded, quite a few of these new topical treatments actually *do* something, and not all of them cost more than $100 an ounce. They contain powerful ingredients like stem cells, growth factors from neonatal foreskins, and plasma—components that have been scientifically proven to improve the skin's texture and generate cell turnover. Cosmeceutical developers have also figured out ways to deliver these active ingredients to that area deep below the epidermis and the dermis—the nexus where the markers of aging start and where intervention can make a huge difference in the signs of aging on the skin's surface. So it's worth a little extra research to sort out the hype from the potions that really do pack a punch. It's yet another way we can take control of our aging process and use cutting-edge science to deliver the best "New Natural" results.

SHOPPING LIST

No one particular product corresponds to a particular age group. Everyone's skin ages at its own pace. But a general rule of thumb is to focus more on protection and cell turnover when you are in your teens and twenties. Then, as you approach 30 and see more signs of aging, bring out the big guns that can work in the deepest layers to rebuild volume, improve elasticity, stimulate

When it comes to cleansing skin, less is more. We North Americans tend to overdo it. When you're in your teens and your skin is more oily and prone to breakouts, or if it's a hot and sticky day, washing your face three or four times a day makes sense, but otherwise you should aim for two cleanses a day. A gentle cleanser is most appropriate for every skin type and age. If you are following my A.M./P.M. regimen, you should already be removing dead skin cells through retinoids, alpha hydroxy acids, and occasional scrubs. Overcleansing is unnecessary and can strip your skin of healthy natural oils and damage the outer layer of the dermis.

stem cells, and give collagen a booster shot. Use rejuvenation products along with antioxidants, sunscreens, and moisturizers daily at any age.

Bear in mind that cosmeceutical companies don't always combine ingredients in a strategic and logical way. Often they will take the latest and most buzz-worthy and shovel them haphazardly into a product line, which almost always consists of a cleanser, a toner, a day moisturizer, a night cream, an eye cream, and sometimes a day and night serum. Most of the time, you don't need to buy the whole product range, so if you are going to splurge on a high-end product, focus on the day and night moisturizers and serums, because they are the ones that will stay on the skin and have the most impact. A good gentle cleanser like Cetaphil will do, while toners really need to be only a basic astringent. And when you shop for these products, look for the ingredients that are most appropriate to use during the day and at night. My rule of thumb is that daytime is all about protection and nighttime is all about renewal. These ingredients don't always belong together. Read the product label carefully and be wary of daytime formulations that combine antioxidants and retinoids, for example. This seems self-defeating to me, considering that retinoids make skin more photosensitive and prone to sun damage. Stick with retinoids for nighttime use only.

Here's a list of skin care ingredients, including a few brands with a cosmeceutical edge that are worth investing in, and brief instructions on how and when to use them:

A.M.:

• Antioxidants: For every age and every day. No exceptions! As I said in Chapter 2, you don't want to go out half-covered. This is an essential component of protection. Apply a nickel-sized amount in the morning, first thing after cleansing, and let the ingredients soak in before you lather up with moisturizer and sunscreen. Sometimes antioxidants come in the form of cleansers and toners, but a serum or moisturizer is best to make sure their protective powers stay with you throughout the day, because they soak in more than cleansers or toners. The latest and greatest scientifically studied antioxidants are polyphenols derived from plants. Look for the following:
  • Catechins: In tea leaves, chocolate, wine.
  • Procyanidins: In grape seed extract.
  • Ferulic acid: In wheat, oats, coffee, apples, spinach. These are commonly added to antioxidant combinations of vitamins C and E.
  • Pomegranate: More powerful than green tea or grape derivatives and shown to improve effectiveness of topical sunscreens.
  • CoffeeBerry: Has 10 times the power of green tea and is also effective in reviving stressed skin. Revale Skin and PRIORI are two skin care lines that contain the ingredient, and more brands are likely to follow suit.
  • Genistein (soy) and Pycnogenol (pine extract): Decreases pigmentation, augments the use of sunscreens, and accelerates wound healing.
  • Biocell SOD (superoxide dismutase): A superpotent enzyme-based antioxidant/free radical scavenger that provides anti-inflammatory and antioxidant effects while offering a layer of protection for the skin.
  • Uniprotect PT-3: A bioactive complex that works at a molecular level to help protect skin proteins from UV-induced oxidation, stimulate the synthesis of repairing enzymes, and accelerate protein repair.

• Moisturizers: Create an optimal environment for skin healing and cell turnover. You need these agents to hydrate and maintain the integrity of your skin. By hydrating the skin and preventing water loss, you improve its barrier against daily environmental stresses and toxins. There are three types of moisturizers, and one kind is more appropriate than another depending upon your skin type and particular issues.

- Emollients: If you have sensitive skin or eczema, go for a light emollient moisturizing agent like octyl octanoate, sesame oil, grape seed oil, or cetyl stearate, which fill in the cracks between cells, soothe the skin, and give it a good "slip" feel. Curél, Eucarin, Moisturel, Aquaphor, and Cetaphil, available at most drugstores, will do the trick. The fewer the perfumes and chemicals, the better.

- Occlusives: If you have psoriasis, go for an occlusive moisturizing agent such as petrolatum, lanolin, mineral oil, and silicones. Apply immediately after bathing or washing your face to trap additional moisture in the skin.

- Humectants: For those with normal skin. They soak in easily without that greasy feel. They work by attracting and binding water to the skin and can penetrate into deeper layers. Humectant ingredients can include propylene glycol, glycerin, urea, hyaluronic acid, Na-PCA, and (this is a mouthful) pyrrolidone carboxylate. Too much humectant can dry the skin, however, so look for a product that contains both an emollient and a humectant. Moisturizers may also be combined with other ingredients, including antioxidants, niacin, panthenol, peptides, and aloe vera. A multitasking moisturizer is fine to use; just be sure to match the task to the problem. And when you are younger, you don't need a heavy cream. A light lotion or gel-based formula will suffice because your skin still produces plenty of its own natural oils and a heavy, oil-based cream could cause breakouts. You also don't have to spend a fortune on a good moisturizer. The key ingredients are basically the same whether you are buying a drugstore brand or something more upscale. Remember that most moisturizers don't stay on the skin for 24 hours, so you need to apply two or three times a day to keep them working for you.

There have been some new and exciting developments in the science of delivering moisturizing agents to skin cells on a continuous, 24-hour basis. Consider these:

BEAUTY ON A BUDGET

Many highly effective and affordable skin care products are available, from the dollar store to the department store. However, there are also home alternatives that often don't require even a shopping trip. Not only do these DIY alternatives work, they are also fun and simple to create.

Calm Acne—Acne can be one of those persistent problems that always seem to pop up at the worst time. We've all had these flare-ups before a big party or an important date. The best at-home treatment for acne is a warm compress: a simple washcloth soaked in some warm water.

Then follow these steps:

1. Apply the compress to the pimple or acne-prone area and hold on for 3 to 5 minutes, warming it up as necessary to maintain a warm feeling on your skin. Be sure not to use water that is too hot. Not only will it burn you, it won't do any good in treating the acne.
2. Repeat the compress every 2 to 4 hours until the acne disappears. Depending on where you are in the breakout, your skin should clear up within 24 to 36 hours.

For an inexpensive product that can be used in conjunction with this remedy, I suggest any acne treatment that contains salicylic acid, benzoyl peroxide, sulfur, and/or resorcinol.

Unclog Blackheads—Not many faces are completely blackhead-free. To help rid your skin of them, mix equal parts oatmeal and rose water to create a soft paste, cover problem areas, and rub in small circular motions, then leave on as you would a face mask. Wait 15 to 20 minutes and then rinse away. You can use this oatmeal mask anytime to give your face a radiant glow. To purchase a comparable product, simply head to your nearest drugstore for Neutrogena Healthy Skin and Neutrogena Healthy Skin Anti-Wrinkle Anti-Blemish Scrub.

Cleanse and Exfoliate—For an affordable and effective skin cleanser and exfoliator, I recommend creating a solution of about a tablespoon of sugar and a teaspoon of water. Before applying the solution, open pores by leaving a warm cloth over your face for a few minutes. Then rub the water-and-sugar solution gently into your skin for about a minute and rinse. Your face will be left clean, clear, and refreshed. For a more aggressive exfoliator, mix in sea salt instead of sugar. This can be used to exfoliate your entire body and works great on those annoying rough spots like feet, knees, and elbows. Salt is also an anti-inflammatory and has antiseptic properties, so it can have additional medicinal benefits when used on the skin. Be sure not to overdo it, though.

Occasional manual exfoliation—about once a week—is good, but not on an everyday basis.

Not interested in making your own exfoliator? Pick up St. Ives Apricot Scrub. It's a solid alternative.

Alleviate Dry Skin—Take a quick trip to your pantry and pull out a bottle of olive oil. Olive oil was good enough for the ancient Greeks to bathe in and to moisturize with, and it's also great for you. Almost every vegetable oil is compatible with the skin. Apply a palm-sized amount of oil daily just after bathing and smooth on gently with your hands to help reduce dry patches and the appearance of stretch marks.

Hydrate—Drink at least four 8-ounce glasses of water every day. We know it's good for us in every way. It makes your skin look great, too.

Nourish—A homemade honey mask is a great way to brighten and lighten the skin on your face. Beat an egg yolk, add 1 teaspoon of olive oil, and blend well. Add 1 tablespoon of honey with a spoon that has been rinsed in hot water and blend the mixture again. Apply this honey mask to your face, avoiding your eye area. Leave on for 20 to 30 minutes and rinse. The improvement in your skin will be visible. Check online for other home facial masks to address your different concerns, whether it's oily skin, dry skin, a combination, or sensitive skin. A great drugstore alternative to the honey mask is the Original Mint Julep Masque.

Tone and Tighten—Witch hazel, also available at any drugstore, is the main ingredient in most toners and works great on its own. Apply it with a cotton ball after washing and drying your face. If you have dry, flaky skin, try diluting the witch hazel with two parts water. Since witch hazel is an astringent, always moisturize after you tone. For a more refreshing toner, try mixing 2 tablespoons of witch hazel with 1 teaspoon of lemon juice and 3 tablespoons of rose water. Always keep witch hazel at home; not only does it do a great job of toning and tightening your skin, it's also an excellent topical remedy for the treatment of traumatic bruises and bumps, and it promotes speedy healing.

Moisturize—Moisturizing is essential for your skin because it locks in hydration and creates a protective barrier between your skin and nature's elements. Making an effective moisturizer at home is not difficult. Put 5 to 6 drops of sweet almond oil in one of your palms and add a few drops of water. Mix the two ingredients in your palms, rubbing both hands together, then gently smooth the blend into your skin. Moisturizing is the bottom line in skin care—almost any moisturizer will do the trick. Eucerin Extra Protective Moisture Lotion with SPF is a great product readily available nationwide.

(continued)

Beauty on a Budget *(continued)*

Soothe—From time to time you may find your skin is red and irritated, and taking care of it at home is as easy as a glass of milk. It doesn't matter if you prefer cow's or soy milk—both get the job done. Soak a washcloth in milk that's cool or room temperature and then apply the cloth to the affected area, pressing gently on the skin for at least 5 minutes. Repeat as often as necessary depending on the irritation. Milk soothes, softens, and nourishes the skin and helps to promote healing. For the store-bought alternative, try an aloe vera gel.

Minimize Pores—Our pores are an open target. They collect oil and often get clogged, causing them to appear larger than we want. To minimize pores for free, run hot water into a stopped sink or a large bowl, then drape a towel over your head and lean over the rising steam for 2 to 3 minutes. Follow this by gently cleansing or exfoliating the skin to help minimize the appearance of clogged pores. Pat skin dry and use a toner to tighten and refine. Neutrogena Pore Minimizing Mask and Bioré Deep Cleansing Pore Strips are excellent over-the-counter pore-minimizing products.

- Aquaporins—Proteins embedded in the cell membrane that regulate the delivery of water. Aquaporin stimulators such as gluco-glycerol get the moisturizing agents delivered through microchannels beneath the surface of the skin and between the skin cells, really keeping the moisture moving through your skin all day. Eucarin, Dior (Dior HydrAction), and Decleor use this new technology. Several other cosmetics companies, including Procter & Gamble, are also about to unleash new moisturizers based on the science of aquaporins. This will soon be the gold standard for keeping skin hydrated and protected throughout the day.

- Aquaxyl—Another ingredient that helps cells maintain moisture and prevents the skin from becoming dehydrated and damaged. Researchers have found that Aquaxyl not only replenishes moisture, but helps the body learn to naturally retain that moisture over time. Cell water loss was reduced after 1 month of using Aquaxyl on the skin.

- Detoxifying agents: These take protection several proactive steps beyond antioxidants. Scientists have recently discovered that you can detoxify and cleanse your cells by stimulating the enzyme proteasome, which breaks down the oxidized proteins that can occur in stressed or aged skin. Alpha longoza, amino lumine, phaeodactylum algae extract, and tocopherol are among the key ingredients to look for in moisturizers and skin serums designed to stimulate proteasomes. Korres has products with detoxifying agents, and Silab is developing products that target proteasomes. Dior's Capture Totale One Essential Skin Boosting Super Serum uses a patented longoza complex to repair damaged cells and recharge proteasome activity. You will likely find more of these ingredients turning up in your antioxidant and moisturizing products in the near future, and they should become a standard in your four-pronged approach to daytime skin protection, particularly if you are older and more prone to cell damage.

P.M.:

• Retinoids: I hope by now I have already driven home the importance of using products with retinoids/retinols and alpha hydroxy creams for cell turnover, a regimen that can begin in your twenties and must continue as you age. We like Retin-A, Renova, Avage, Tazorac, and Differin. Many other brands contain these ingredients, and if you are prone to redness and irritation, choose something in a lower strength. Use at least twice a week, at night, alternate with other topicals, and give your skin a chance to calm down between treatments. Topical retinol products really work. One of our patients noticed measurable results after 8 weeks of using one: wrinkle length around her eyes was reduced by *half!*

• Peptides: When you start to notice that your skin isn't as taut and smooth as it was when you were 25, you know it's time to break out the peptide and protein derivatives. Gravity takes its toll on the aging face, but protein and copper peptides stimulate collagen production, which is essential to restoring elasticity in the skin. When collagen is broken down, short segments of three to five amino acids form that are called peptides. These "miniproteins" are active molecules that signal to your skin it was damaged and needs to make new

Many of these topicals are expensive, especially those brands with the newest patented ingredients. So do yourself a favor and give each product a chance to work. It takes 6 to 8 weeks to see a noticeable difference. The damage didn't occur overnight, and neither will its reversal. Also, be consistent about use. Follow the application directions or the advice of your dermatologist, and persist before you give up or decide the product is not working for you.

collagen. Applying peptides topically at least once a day is a way to trick your skin into thinking that it has lost collagen recently and needs to make more. The nice thing about peptides is that they are minuscule and come in light formulations for easy absorption, so they can soak deep into the living layers of the skin at the dermis level and revive cells from the bottom up. Look for palmitoyl pentapeptide-3 (Matrixyl), which is one of the most common ingredients in the latest range of skin care products, including the affordable Oil of Olay's Regenerist, Avon's Anew, and the more expensive brand Stri-Vectin, among many others. Another option is SYN-Coll, a small peptide proven to reduce wrinkles and boost collagen production. Also consider copper peptides, which promote collagen production, work as antioxidants, and act as healing agents by delivering copper deep into the skin. Copper has been used for centuries to heal wounds. It helps remove damaged collagen and replaces it with new, skin-tightening collagen. Neutrogena's Visibly Firm Night Cream and Neova Copper Peptide Complex feature copper peptides.

• Skin brighteners: Most of us experience some form of excess skin pigmentation—freckles, blotches, discoloration—as we age, and using lightening agents helps to restore the overall luminosity of the skin that is a subtle marker of youth. But lightening agents have gotten a bad rap lately with stories about Michael Jackson whitening his skin and disaster cases of women in Asian cultures bleaching and disfiguring themselves in the quest to look whiter. That's not the point of a skin brightener, which functions to even skin tone and reverse pigmentation caused by sun damage. The best-known ingredient in these types of products is hydroquinone, which has been used to regulate pigment production for the past 45 years. The FDA has warned of some cancer risk if you use this product in very large amounts, but I believe that for cosmetic purposes, there's no way you would ever use enough of the active ingredient to create a problem. If you are nervous, however, there are new, non-hydroquinone products available that work with comparable efficacy, including Lumixyl, a physician-dispensed lotion that contains a synthetic peptide developed by dermatologists to improve pigmentation. We've seen good results with the product in our research lab. Avon's Anew and Neutrogena's Ageless Intensives are other skin care lines with formulations to safely correct skin tone. I also like Avon Solutions Neck & Chest Perfector, which evens out skin tone and prevents age spots from forming in the first place. Other agents that work on skin tone are derived from vitamin B, niacin, and nicotinamide, as well as soy and shiitake mushrooms, which are not as strong. Skin care companies are all working on the next effective hydroquinone substitute. Sepiwhite has also proven effective as an age spot fader that helps to control hyperpigmentation. Sepiwhite helps maintain skin integrity and reduces the synthesis of melanin pigments. It has also been shown to inhibit melanogenesis caused by UV radiation. Kojic acid is a widely used, proven whitener and skin brightener. Also consider licorice root extracts or licorice PTH, a specially purified extract of licorice root with a high percentage of the glabridin component. These are effective in inhibiting melanin production, which is responsible for the dark pigmentation of the skin. Alternate skin brighteners with retinoids and alpha hydroxy acids. If you're using all three, use each twice a week. You should see improvement in about 2 months.

• Anti-inflammatories: Redness or flushing is another sign of aging, although the problem of rosacea is not exclusive to my older patients. One of the best ways to treat this condition, which worsens over time, is to zap it with intense pulsed light lasers to shrink the supply of blood to the blood vessels. But dermatological science has recently discovered new cosmeceutical ingredients that act as lasers in a jar: alpha longoza, licorice, phytosphingosine, aloe vera, and soy derivatives. Studies we published in the *Journal of Drugs in Dermatology* discuss the significant decline in redness people experienced when they used these cosmeceuticals, almost on a par with the results of an IPL treatment. Alpha longoza, which I have already mentioned a few times in this book because of its striking efficacy, is the extract of the rare longoza fruit. It is particularly potent and doubles as a growth factor to regenerate cells. It can be found in high concentrations in Dior's Capture line. Other brands use licorice extract among other calming ingredients like aloe. This is an area of cosmeceuticals that's poised to really take off with the recent discovery of what these extracts can do. Phytosphingosine is another ingredient that is highly effective at reducing acne, redness, and inflammation and can inhibit the growth of microorganisms on the skin, resulting in smaller, less visible pores.

• Growth factors, stem cell modulators, gene-boosting technology, sirtuin activators, and signaling molecules called cytokines: These all improve cell survival and cause your cells to produce new proteins. I am so excited about this new frontier in skin care that I have dedicated all of Chapter 8 to stem cells and their related components, so I'll talk about them just briefly for now. Many of the newest cosmeceuticals have increasing concentrations of growth factors, or the signaling molecules that can stimulate the biological effects that normally occur in healthy young skin. SkinMedica is a promising new line of cosmeceuticals that contains multiple human growth factors derived from stem cell (i.e., neonatal foreskin) banks that have been clinically studied and found to reduce wrinkles and improve volume and elasticity. More recently, Dior has patented a technology used in its Capture Totale and Capture XP range called Stemsone that keeps existing skin stem cells alive for longer. Stem cells are primitive cells that are actively reproducing all the time. Adult stem cells can't live in a topical skin care product; however, scientists have developed stem cell modulators that do target and protect preexisting stem cells living on the skin and enable them to be active for a longer period of time, in effect counteracting the normal aging process. There are several skin care products out there with molecules that stimulate cell, collagen, and vascular growth, and you'll recognize them on the ingredients list by these initials:

TGFB, BFGF, and VEGF. Other growth factors to look out for are sirtuin activators such as resveratrol, kluyveromyces yeast biopeptides, *Aframomum angustifolium,* and *Malva sylvestris.* Sirtuins are master genes that function at the epidermis, the dermis, and the epidermal/dermal junction known as the aging responsible interface—the area that regulates elasticity, wrinkles, discoloration, and other age markers. We don't have the nanotechnology to put sirtuins in skin care products yet, but like the stem cell modulators, the sirtuin activators help stimulate and protect your sirtuins and prolong the life expectancy of those living cells deep beneath the surface. When we studied all of these growth factors and stem cell modulators in our labs, we saw a significant reduction of wrinkles in patients who used these formulations twice a day for 2 months. Collagen in the 14 women who participated in the clinical study increased by 37 percent, and epidermal thickening increased by 30 percent. Wrinkling around the eyes was reduced by about 70 percent over 6 months. L'Oréal's newest anti-aging line called Youth Code claims to harness gene-boosting technology. As science evolves and we have a greater understanding of biology, more and more products will include advanced scientific solutions based on cutting-edge science. This is an exciting new world for all of us.

* **If you wish to know more about these ingredients, their cosmeceutical efficacy has been scientifically legitimized through our clinically published studies in the *Journal of Drugs in Dermatology* and my new medical book, *Cosmeceutical Science in Clinical Practice* [London: Informa Healthcare, 2010].**

CUSTOM-BUILD

There are so many ingredients and products out there, which ones should you use? Well, I can't answer that question for you entirely. A skin care regimen should be built around your particular needs and concerns. Ideally, you will have discussed and defined your problems with your dermatologist, who can then give you guidelines about what to look for at the cosmetics counter and help you decide which ingredients are best for your particular skin issues and whether or not certain pricey compounds are even necessary. If you are spending lots of money on a new product, you are entitled to ask for samples to test it out before you make the investment, to make sure it doesn't have a perfume or emollient that irritates your skin. You should also like the way it feels and be happy with how it smells so that you will want to use it.

Once you have your skin care arsenal assembled, you should think in terms of building blocks. You'll have the products you cannot do without—the sunscreens, antioxidants, and retinoids. You'll probably have two types of moisturizer—one with daytime ingredients and the other with nighttime renewal formulations. Then you'll add on and occasionally alternate the specialty treatments, such as peptides, skin brighteners, and compounds to help with rosacea, or stem cell modulators for wrinkle repair. Divide your regimen into A.M. and P.M., and layer each product, leaving a minute or two for each compound to soak in before you add the next building block. Once you begin to understand the role of each ingredient, your regimen will make perfect sense to you and will hopefully become as automatic as combing your hair in the morning.

IDIOT-PROOF

You can also ask your dermatologist to custom-blend formulations for your own skin. These days, most dermatologists even have a ready-made skin care line sitting on the shelves of their office waiting rooms. The advantage to using these products is that you can get both prescription-strength ingredients and the regular oversight of a specialist who can make necessary adjustments along the way. Think of it as "idiot-proofing" your skin care regimen.

Adam, my chief of operations, went this route and now at 37 looks better than he did when he joined Sadick Dermatology 7 years ago. And we have thousands of patients with the same results.

Let's use Adam as our example. He looks a little like a clean-shaven version of the fashion designer Tom Ford. But he wasn't making the most of his good looks. Long Island born and raised, he'd spent a few too many summers sun worshipping at the beach. His Mediterranean skin was sallow, there was too much freckling and pigmentation, and he looked tired and stressed from working long hours as a business and marketing consultant. I would never have guessed he was 30 when I first met him. And since he would be the very public face of Sadick Dermatology, promoting my practice and business interests, we needed to do better by him. But I'll let Adam tell you the rest in his own words:

As a guy, I am very low maintenance. I guess I never really thought about the importance of taking care of my skin. At most, my routine was a little soap and water in the shower. And I was bad about using sunscreen. As a kid, I never burned. I took my olive skin for granted. But in my twenties I did start to burn, and by my 30th birthday, I realized I could no longer get away with it. Luckily, I found myself in the right place at the right time.

Dr. Sadick put me on an A.M./P.M. regimen. In the morning, I started using a rejuvenation compound that's a cocktail of every anti-aging, anti-oxidant ingredient you can imagine. For night, he gave me a prescription-strength moisturizer that contained a combination of glycolic acid for cell turnover and a skin brightener, hydroquinone, to even out my skin tone and reverse all those years of sun damage. He also gave me a light gly-colic cleanser to keep the occasional acne breakout in check.

It's a stepped program, and each prescription formulation goes from 1 to 4 in strength levels. The idea is to keep skin stimulated. You use level 1 for a few months to a year, see what the skin tolerates, and when you're ready to go to the next level, you move up the chain.

It was a subtle change, and people started noticing the improvement before I did. They'd comment that I looked rested, but I certainly wasn't getting any more sleep than usual. Then, after about 6 months, I noticed a gradual improvement in the tone and texture of my skin. The freckles were almost gone. The surface of my face was smooth. I'd forgotten what healthy skin was supposed to look like, and then the luminosity came back. There's [now] a plumpness and moisture to the skin that catches the light in a certain way and makes me look more alive.

The great thing about this program is that the improvement is continual. When I realize I am starting to plateau, I check in with Dr. Sadick and he moves me to the next level. I can honestly say that at 37 I have no lines on my face, not even the slightest feathery wrinkle around my eyes, and I am convinced this is due to the skin care routine that's become automatic to me. Sure, I've done a couple of minor procedures: a little Botox now and then; some Sculptra filler to replace lost volume in my cheeks. Working for one of the world's top dermatologists, how could I not? But these treatments don't explain the quality and thickness of my skin's surface.

Using prescription topicals has been the biggest change to my regimen. The best part is that I don't have to think about it. I just grab one bottle in the morning and another bottle at night. It takes seconds to apply and I'm done. I know they are the best ingredients, they have been chosen for a reason in consultation with my doctor, and they actually do something for me. My goal is not to look younger than my age, but to look good for my age. Having healthy-looking skin is the key to achieving my goal. I know I look good for my age, and with Dr. Sadick's advice and products, I always will.

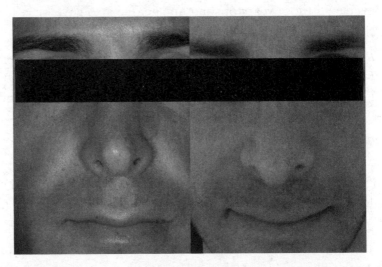

Tighter pores, more even skintone, and improved volume make Adam's skin look at least five years younger than it did seven years ago.

Adam's right. If he sticks to his regimen, he will continue to look young and healthy for whatever decade he is in. The older we get, the slower the dermis regenerates itself and repairs the damage, but the extraordinary over-the-counter and prescription compounds I have mentioned will give your skin the booster shot it needs to maintain that youthful glow. The trick is knowing what to look for on the list of active ingredients. And remember, your skin doesn't stop at the jawline. Don't forget to use the same products you would use on your face—sunblocks, antioxidants, moisturizers, peptides, retinols, and others—on your neck, chest, and even your hands—all the places that show signs of aging.

Today's list of cosmeceuticals is long, complex, and growing, but there is truly something for everyone, from expensive designer brands to creams you can find for less than $20 at your nearest Walgreens. And if you use them correctly and consistently, you can sustain your youthful looks long enough to forestall a trip to your dermatologist's office for stronger and more expensive anti-aging interventions. They can be part of an easy daily maintenance regimen that doesn't necessarily have to cost a fortune and will make all the difference in preventing or minimizing the ravages of time on your skin.

CHAPTER SIX

FROM THE INSIDE OUT

YOU ARE WHAT YOU EAT, SOME OF THE TIME

Any natural cosmetic regimen must include diet and nutrition, yet I almost resisted writing about it. Not only is there a glut of books out there on nutrition and its effect on overall health and appearance, but the topic itself is often overdiscussed. While it's undoubtedly healthy to eat oatmeal for breakfast and salmon for dinner and snack on antioxidant-rich berries in between, there's little scientific evidence to suggest this kind of diet will do anything to reverse existing wrinkles. Truth be told, no one ever "ate" their way to beauty. It's not that simple.

I know this goes against convention. Diet and exercise are paramount to health and fitness, and obviously the better you look, the better you feel; and the better you feel, the better you look—at least to some extent. All the cosmetic procedures in the world won't make much of a difference to your quality of life if you're unhealthy, malnourished, or out of shape. That being said, good nutrition and health certainly facilitate recovery and repair following a cosmetic procedure, and bad habits like drinking and smoking to excess can impede the re-formation of collagen. As an internist as well as a dermatologist, I always encourage my patients to adopt healthy habits well before they undergo a procedure. Healing could always use some extra help from the right amount of nutrients.

But once you have sun damage or wrinkles or sagging, the right diet is not going to make them go away. How we age has more to do with our genetics, our exposure to sun and environmental damage, and the preventive and regenerative topical regimens we follow every day. I know plenty of women who are not health-conscious when it comes to their diet but still look amazing for their decade. Conversely, there are women who are fit, count every calorie, and balance every meal yet look every bit their age, if not older. Sure, in extreme cases of poor nutrition, symptoms are going to show on your skin, just as the wrong diet can exacerbate immunologic disorders and cause external symptoms. But for the rest of us, the relationship between what we put in our mouths and what happens to our skin is not that direct.

NUTRIENT SATURATION

All that said, we're discovering a wealth of new antioxidants, nutrients, and compounds that can protect and, to some degree, regenerate our cells. While most of these ingredients may be more effective when applied externally as a cream or serum, it stands to reason that they could offer an additional boost from the inside out. Why not stack the deck in your favor by taking in extra nutrients and antioxidants? It's not necessarily going to fix a preexisting problem, but at the very least, you will avoid potential nutrient depletion and promote healthy cells over the long term.

The skin recuperation process slows as we age, so the act of saturating the body with the necessary micro- and macronutrients is essential if we want the healing process to operate at maximum efficiency. Skin is one of the most powerful indicators of health and youth, so taking care of yourself on the inside with proper nutrition and lifestyle can greatly impact your appearance on the outside. This is something that cannot be faked, covered up, or corrected. And the better your skin looks naturally, the better it will look after any cosmetic procedure.

So let's address what we really need to know about using nutrition to enhance our looks.

THE BASICS

All foods are made up of macronutrients and micronutrients. There are only three macronutrients: protein, fats, and carbohydrates; and all foods contain one, two, or all three of them. When it comes to eating right for your skin, protein and fats are the most essential to healing, especially when you are recovering from a cosmetic procedure like liposuction or laser skin resurfacing. Protein sources repair cells and build new ones, and fats provide suppleness, moisture, and elasticity to skin. Make sure you are getting enough of both. Carbohydrates are basically an energy source with little direct effect on tissue, so they should be eaten in moderation. I know there are numerous suggestions out there regarding the proper ratio of protein, fats, and carbs to consume at each meal, but I recommend simply observing a balance. No single meal should be just pasta or just meat. There's no need for complex, preplanned meal programs. Just use variety and a little common sense.

The best protein sources for your skin are lean meats, fish, chicken, and eggs. Vegetable protein such as soy and nuts are fine, but they do not contain all the essential amino acids necessary for completing the protein chain required for collagen production. Without protein, nothing can grow or repair itself. Your skin also needs fat, but people fear fat for two reasons: They equate it with body fat and the clogging of arteries. However, the key to maintaining a healthy body and healthy skin is to consume heart-healthy, unsaturated fats like olive oil at every meal and keep the nasty saturated fats like butter to a minimum. Olive oil has been used in beauty treatments for years to give skin and hair a nice luster. Fish oils are also great for you: They contain the coveted omega-3 fatty acids that have been known to protect against heart disease, and over time, in combination with other good habits, they can give skin a smooth, velvety glow.

Though it contains no vitamins or macro elements, fiber is a compound that benefits our health by clinging to food and helping in its elimination, keeping us regular and "cleansed." Sluggish digestion can lead to a buildup of toxins that can appear on our skin in the form of acne and inflammation. But don't fall for the claim that fiber is the answer to staying thin and looking beautiful. Yes, it contains almost no calories and fills us up and has an indirect beauty benefit, but it is void of nutrition and too much can cause digestive distress. As in everything else to do with damage prevention and skin maintenance, it is about balance.

KNOW YOUR A, C, E'S

The other elements in food that may help your skin are micronutrients. Micronutrients are the vitamins, minerals, and enzymes present in foods that have a healing and revitalizing component. On top of the list for collagen production is vitamin C. Without vitamin C, tissue fibers become less elastic, which will lead to sagging skin. Vitamin C also protects against free radical damage—a huge contributor to premature skin aging. There is an abundance of research on vitamin C, starting with the eminent American chemist who was among the first to realize its importance: Linus Pauling, PhD. Back in 1986, Dr. Pauling concluded: "A person who is dying of scurvy [which vitamin C cures] stops making this substance, and his body falls apart—his joints fail, because he can no longer keep the cartilage and tendons strong, his blood vessels break open, his gums ulcerate and his teeth fall out, his immune system deteriorates." Dr. Pauling goes on to explain how collagen is one of thousands of different kinds of proteins in the human body: "Collagen as strong white fibers, stronger than steel wire of the same weight, and as yellow elastic networks . . . constitutes the connective tissue that holds our bodies together." That analysis was incredibly astute for Dr. Pauling's time, and over the years he has been proven correct. Vitamin C is one of our greatest allies in the fight against aging.[6]

Two key companions of vitamin C are bioflavonoids and rutin. Both are present in foods containing vitamin C. Bioflavonoids are a part of plant pigments with antioxidant, antiallergic, anticarcinogenic, antiviral, and anti-inflammatory properties. Rutin enhances the role of bioflavonoids by acting as a natural detoxifier. It attaches itself to metal ions that are ever-present in our polluted environment and prevents the reactions that form free radicals, which are responsible for skin deterioration. It's also good for the circulatory system, strengthening the capillaries and improving blood flow, which can contribute to our skin's overall radiance.

There's also some evidence that rutin helps maintain levels of collagen in the skin and prevents wrinkling and sun damage. Topically, cosmetic companies have found ways to produce stable versions of vitamin C and its two sidekicks, which make for great antioxidant creams and serums. But as supplements, you'd need to ingest thousands of extra units daily to have a direct impact on the skin. And you'd urinate most of that extra dosage out of your system before it could do much good anyway. Better to stick to the recommended daily levels that already exist in a healthy diet and let your body do the rest.

Research shows that vitamin E is also a potent antioxidant that helps reduce the harmful effects of the sun on the skin. According to studies published by the American Academy of Dermatology, taking 400 units of vitamin E daily appeared to reduce the risk of sun damage to cells as well as reduce the production of cancer-causing cells.[7] Some studies confirm that when vitamins E and A are taken together, people show a 70 percent reduction in basal cell carcinoma, a common form of skin cancer. So of all the nutrients, vitamin E probably has the most direct benefit on the skin. Because it's fat soluble and, unlike vitamin C, doesn't get flushed away quickly through urine, vitamin E sticks around in the body long enough to reach the epidermis and provide antioxidant benefits to skin cells.[7] Vitamin E is also a blood thinner, which is why it is not recommended prior to surgery (to avoid excess bleeding). But for nonsurgical procedures, there are no complications from vitamin E, and it will aid in recovery and the prevention of bruising.

Also critical to skin quality is vitamin A, which allows for the regeneration and tissue repair of all the cells in the body, particularly skin cells. As already discussed in Chapter 3, a topical version, Retin-A, is based on the molecular structure of vitamin A and has been proven to have a corrective effect on skin damage and fine wrinkles. Vitamin A also forms the basis for Accutane, a common treatment for severe acne because it can decrease the size of sebaceous glands and the amount of oil they produce. While it has less direct impact on the skin when taken internally, adequate vitamin A is imperative to healthy, vibrant skin tone as well as vision and bone health. But that does not mean you should rush out to the vitamin store to buy an economy-sized jar of vitamin A supplements. Western diets already provide plenty of vitamin A, which is available in abundance in carrots, sweet potatoes, spinach, broccoli, liver, kale, red peppers, and mangoes and to a lesser degree in most other fruits and vegetables. Topically, yes, buy a retinoid, but foodwise, a few carrots in your salad are plenty!

INNER STRENGTH

Flavonoids, polyphenols, resveratrol: The list of skin-boosting antioxidants derived from food and plants is forever growing. One relative newcomer to the skin care industry is the extensively researched coenzyme Q10 (CoQ10), which has at least two important functions in the body. First, it acts as an antioxidant, neutralizing harmful free radicals, which are one of the causes of aging. Second, CoQ10 is an essential cog in the machinery that produces biological energy (known as ATP, or adenosine triphosphate—the substance that allows muscles and skin to contract) inside the cells. This energy is imperative when recovering from a procedure such as a filler injection or an ablative (skin-injuring) laser treatment because it can accelerate the healing process.

Though CoQ10 occurs naturally in the body, various factors such as aging, stress, and some types of medication can lower its effectiveness and, consequently, jeopardize the ability of cells to withstand stress and regenerate. In some studies, rodents treated with supplemental CoQ10 lived up to 30 percent longer than their untreated counterparts and maintained youthful behavior longer. CoQ10 taken as a supplement or applied topically may boost skin repair and reduce free radical damage. A good dosage is between 10 and 100 milligrams a day.

PLANT POWER

Another way to protect your skin against the harmful effects of sun and the environment is by taking in flavonoid phytochemicals, or polyphenols—the antioxidants found in great abundance in green tea. Numerous studies have shown that green tea polyphenols can help reduce inflammation, fight infections, and even prevent cardiovascular disease and certain cancers. The data are less conclusive on its benefits to the skin, but there is enough anecdotal evidence to suggest it may be worth making a habit of drinking green tea throughout the day. Animal studies have indicated some sun protection benefit from green tea, and a couple of small human studies suggest its anti-inflammatory effects can help control rosacea and improve skin elasticity in photoaged skin. I would recommend drinking 3 to 10 cups per day or taking a green tea supplement of 300 milligrams twice per day.

Resveratrol, another plant-derived antioxidant found in the skin of red grapes and in wine, packs even more of a punch than green tea. The buzz about resveratrol turned into a siren call recently when scientists figured out a way to produce a stabilized form of it, which has been shown in some studies to activate sirtuins, a class of enzyme that is partly responsible for regulating cell defense and promoting longevity. Early studies suggest that taken internally, resveratrol can help prevent lung, breast, and colon cancers and lower blood sugar. And resveratrol is one of the few nutrients that probably does more good when ingested than when applied as a topical, because the ingredient tends to oxidize when exposed to the air. Studies remain to be done, but that's not going stop me from taking my twice daily dose of 60 milligrams!

I know it's a lot to digest. Trying to negotiate all the foods and combinations of foods involved in obtaining these nutrients practically requires a degree in biochemistry, and this is where some people get discouraged. But instead of becoming a slave to a lengthy list of foods high in specific vitamins, there's an easier solution. You cannot beat a good basic "one a day" multivitamin pill. Most have more vitamin C, for example, than a hundred oranges. You may wonder, "Aren't food sources better?" Well, yes and no. Food has some factors that assist each micronutrient in doing its job, but when it comes to actual vitamin C and most of the other essential nutrients, the body merely recognizes the molecule (which a multivitamin provides). And some of the better synthetic vitamin formulas also contain helpful vitamin C cofactors such as rutin and the bioflavonoids that occur naturally in fruits and vegetable. You should look at the list of any vitamin supplement to make sure they're included.

There are lots of other easy ways to make up for a less than stellar diet. A protein shake is a nutrient-dense meal without loads of calories, though some are better than others. Whey protein is preferable to soy protein; because of the amino acid complex issue, vegetable proteins are less complete. And instead of buying expensive pre-made protein drinks, you can buy protein powder directly from the factory online and make your own milkshakes and smoothies. They'll taste better, and you'll have more control over what goes into them.

Naturally, vitamin supplements should never be used as an alternative to a healthy diet, but they can provide nutrient saturation, which is next to impossible to obtain from food alone. A new twist on the skin supplement is a type of health drink called the nutracosmeceutical. Yes, it's a mouthful, both linguistically and literally. The Japanese were among the first to develop nutracosmeceuticals based on the idea that the more you can pack into a beverage to target a certain skin issue, the better. They are filled with antioxidants, moisturizing ingredients, skin whiteners, and cell boosters. They claim to firm skin and erase lines with their amino acids, peptides, proteins, and, in some Japanese versions, hyaluronic acid. Nutracosmeceuticals are starting to make their way onto American drugstore shelves. One product line I've seen in the skin care section is Borba Skin Balance Water. Touting itself as "drinkable skin care," it contains exotic ingredients like pomegranate extract as well as vitamins like C and E. But, again, there's very little science to support the claims that what you take in will show up externally in these specific ways. Sure, it's a good idea in theory, but mostly it's another way for enterprising dermatologists to brand themselves and make money. There's no harm in buying these drinks, but they are expensive (a 12-pack of Borba Skin Balance Water costs about $25). If you can afford it and want to give it a try, go for it. Just don't expect any miracles.

TOO MUCH OF A GOOD THING

It's hard to take in enough of these ingredients to show up on your skin, and it's not always wise to try. When it comes to nutrients, more isn't always better. A little extra is okay, but certain vitamins such as A and E are stored in body fat, and too much could result in buildup and possible liver toxicity.

Vitamin C, on the other hand, is water soluble, meaning whatever we don't use passes through the urine. For this reason, we need a constant supply of vitamin C and overdose is virtually impossible. If any vitamin should be taken in addition to a multivitamin formula, it should be vitamin C. Take 500 milligrams in the morning and another 500 milligrams midday. If you are recovering from even a mildly invasive procedure, I'd recommend yet another 500 milligrams at bedtime.

As for the rest of your nutrient intake, simply stick to a balanced diet, with emphasis on protein and vegetables. As much as possible, forgo refined and processed foods like white bread and pasta in complex carbohydrates like whole grains, to keep inflammation in check.

THE EXTRAS

A few other recently identified nutrients may also be good for the skin. They occur naturally in the body, but because they don't quite fall into the "food source" category, you can derive additional benefits by taking them in supplement form. One nutrient directly related to skin quality is hyaluronic acid, which belongs to the class of compounds known as glycosaminoglycans. The connection between the decline in the body's concentration of hyaluronic acid and signs of aging has long been of interest to clinical researchers. Hyaluronic acid is a component of connective tissue that has been touted as a preventive measure for arthritis because of its ability to cushion and lubricate joints, but more recently it's been shown to aid in collagen synthesis. This is one reason hyaluronic acid is among the most popular of the new dermal fillers. Taken internally, a reasonable supplement dosage is between 25 and 50 milligrams a day.

Dimethylaminoethanol (DMAE) has long been regarded as an effective brain booster because of its ability to remove lipofuscin—a form of molecular waste that accumulates in the brain and is thought to be responsible for senility. DMAE occurs naturally in sardines, helping the fish live up to its title of "good brain food," and can also be found in almost any health food store in capsule or tablet form. DMAE may be effective in tightening sagging skin or at least preventing further sag. There is still speculation as to how this works or to what degree, but the skin and health supplement industries have been quick to jump on this latest find and produce more overpriced creams containing DMAE. I am not sure how stable and safe these topicals are, but there may also be beauty benefits to taking DMAE internally. The recommended dosage is 100 milligrams a day.

DRINK UP!

The final component to healthy skin is hydration. Without proper hydration, the skin dries and elastin begins to break down. Nutrition experts, doctors, and other proponents of good hydration also claim that drinking water gives the skin a radiant, healthy, youthful complexion with no wrinkles and allows skin to maintain its elasticity and suppleness. This may be a bit of an overstatement, but it doesn't negate the main message: Drink water, and lots of it!

How about spraying or misting water on the skin to help reduce dryness? Are water treatments, steams, and humidifiers effective? There are significant differences of opinion, but the debate is overblown. I believe it's simply a matter of environment. Moisture-saturated air limits how much escapes from your skin, while dry air draws moisture out. So if you live in a humid environment, you're likely to have more supple skin. If you live in an area where it's dry, or where the winters are cold and you must rely on dry heat, then yes, additional water both internally and externally is recommended.

Drinking water in adequate amounts is also necessary to flush toxins out of the body via the excretory system, and that too has an effect on our skin. If the body suffers from inadequate hydration, these toxins can build up and escape through skin pores, contributing to dry skin, acne, eczema, psoriasis, dark circles around the eyes, fine lines, and wrinkles. By flushing the body internally with water and enabling the toxins to release through the skin, these problems are less likely to occur.

There's also some debate over what *type* of water is best. Some swear that distilled water is the purest, while others think it's essentially "dead" water. You've probably heard people tell horror stories about all the chemicals in tap water. Others will say that bottled water is no better. One expert might recommend a water filter, while another argues that the filter itself gets so clogged, it actually attracts toxins and sediments. Mineral water contains the natural minerals our body needs, but others claim they aren't necessary and may increase sodium retention. I say that as long as the water is clean and tastes good, you needn't worry too much.

How much water to drink is another question that will get you an assortment of answers. There's nothing wrong with the conventional wisdom that you should drink eight 8-ounce glasses of water a day, although it doesn't have a steep basis in science. It is a rule often quoted but difficult to trace back to any medical or scientific study. In my opinion, an average-sized adult with healthy kidneys who is living in a temperate climate really needs only four glasses of water a day to obtain the benefits of drinking water and to replace daily water loss. But since even 10 or 12 glasses won't cause any harm, there's no reason not to have them. Obviously, forcing liquids in the belief that it will "cleanse" the body is foolish, as is fasting or the use of colonics. These are unhealthy practices that are based more on exploiting the average consumer's fear of toxins than on sound science.

Water to hydrate the skin can be obtained from eating water-rich fruits (such as melons) and vegetables. Some evidence suggests that water in food stays in the body longer and thus has a better chance of being absorbed, whereas drinking water itself gets expelled before proper absorption can take place. Beverages such as milk and juice also contribute to daily water intake. Even caffeinated beverages (which are said to dehydrate) are useful, because according to research, the caffeine is more than compensated for by the amount of water in the beverage itself. A cup of coffee actually adds about two-thirds of a cup of hydrating fluid. So drinking a cup of coffee will add to your water intake total. However, alcoholic beverages result in a net loss of water in the body. If you insist on consuming alcohol, supplement it with extra water.

Seltzer is water with carbon dioxide added, and there's some debate as to its hydrating benefit since our bodies expel carbon dioxide. But the amount is slight, and if you enjoy seltzer, I see no problem with drinking it in place of regular water. However, "club" and other sodas contain bicarbonate, which causes constipation, thus defeating the purpose of toxin release. Try to avoid these types of drinks.

When it comes to staying hydrated, listen to your body. If you lack energy, are constantly thirsty, and have dark urine, this could be a sign that you are not getting enough water. Thirst is the body's way of signaling a need to increase water intake. So pay attention to this warning sign. Never go thirsty.

IT ALL HELPS

Keeping these simple nutritional suggestions in mind can make a world of difference in the health and appearance of your skin and in how well you respond to the various procedures you might opt for throughout your life. A single trip to the health food store will cover most, if not all, of your nutrient requirements. It doesn't take a drastic change of behavior; just try to make what you eat a part of your beauty regimen. And swallowing a few supplements in the morning takes less time than putting on some lipstick. No, it won't necessarily reverse existing damage, but it could help prevent or slow more signs of aging.

The jury's still out on how much the consumption of these nutrients and compounds can directly impact the health and appearance of our skin. There needs to be more research, and the beauty and supplement industries overstate many of their claims just to sell more books and products. But, hey, a little more water and a few extra nutrients certainly can't hurt!

CHAPTER SEVEN

THE TOXINS

IF YOU CAN'T FOLD THE PAPER, IT DOESN'T CREASE

I recently saw a patient in her early fifties who had no wrinkles. Not a line. Erica had never had a face-lift, and she'd never tried filler or laser resurfacing. She started getting Botox in her early forties, but never too much. She could still raise her eyebrows and show emotion in her face. It was just enough to hold everything in place, preserve the underlying integrity of her facial muscles, and slow the breakdown of collagen. That and a good skin care regimen made her face almost flawless.

Neurotoxins like Botox are among the most useful tools for maintenance that dermatologists have at their disposal. By decreasing facial expression and minimizing muscle contraction around the areas of the face that are most prone to wrinkles, you can give yourself a tremendous advantage in the fight against aging and keep your skin looking smooth for decades. Botox should not be the only action you take to improve your skin, but as Erica discovered, it is a powerful weapon.

Botox is the brand name for a diluted form of botulinum toxin. It was originally used in the 1960s to treat neurological disorders such as musculo-skeletal spasticity, or muscle spasm, and in 1989 it received FDA approval to treat crossed eyes and blepharospasm (uncontrollable blinking and twitching in the eyes). That's when doctors noticed it also softened frown lines. Botox has also been used off-label to treat migraines, back problems, and excessive sweating. By 1997, it was approved by the FDA for cosmetic use, and since then almost five million cosmetic procedures using Botox and other brands of neurotoxin have been performed. It has become one of the most wildly popular ways to fight the ravages of time.

Botox is excellent for maintaining youth at a later age, but I could just as easily have included this chapter in the prevention section. Ideally, patients should start using Botox or its equivalent at a much younger age than Erica, to decrease dynamic expression well before those fine lines start to appear. If you can't fold the paper, it never creases. In fact, I am seeing more and more women in their twenties using Botox as an age prophylactic. They don't need much, but even a bit softens the fine lines starting to appear, especially on the forehead and around the eyes.

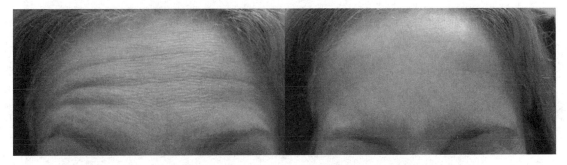

A single treatment of Botox dramatically softened this patient's forehead lines, resulting in a younger appearance.

Common Botox injection sites for erasing wrinkles and lines include the following:

• Glabella (the region between the eyebrows)

• Forehead

- Outer corners of eyes (the wrinkles there are known as crow's-feet)

- Midchin area, to correct lines around the corners of the mouth

- Neck, for those horizontal grooves that can appear across the throat

We also use Botox to treat a few other problems:

- Facial asymmetry or other facial conditions that result from muscle action; this is called facial shaping

- Hyperhidrosis (excessive perspiration); common injection sites include underarms, palms, scalp, and soles of feet

Nostril flaring can be fixed with Botox, but here I urge caution. Be very certain that your physician has used Botox in this way many times, and successfully. This is a controversial application for the neurotoxin, which has been approved by the FDA only for areas around the eyes and forehead. You don't want to risk paralyzing important facial nerves. One false move could cause the sides of your mouth to droop and even affect speech. Seek this kind of Botox treatment only from a professional with significant experience in treating the nose.

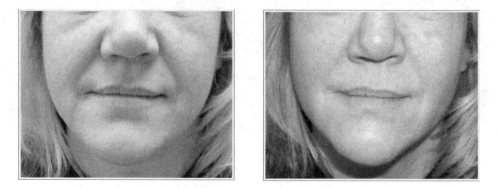

This patient received Botox to soften nostril flaring.

In my practice, we use neurotoxins as part of a multipronged approach to age reversal and prevention. The drug can partially or totally immobilize certain expression muscles in the face that contract and cause wrinkles. It can soften, erase, and prevent wrinkles in the forehead, between the brows, and around the eyes. It can even smooth out neck bands. The effects last for about 120 days, depending on the patient, and the treatment is virtually painless, with no downtime.

Botox costs between $250 and $1,000 per treatment, depending upon your geography, the physician, and the amount of Botox used. Be sure to ask your doctor about the dilution rate. Some practitioners can manipulate cost by diluting Botox. So while you may think you are getting a bargain, your treatment won't be as effective or long lasting if the dosage has been watered down. The introduction of competing toxins, like Dysport, which I consider to be as safe and effective as Botox, will eventually lower the price of these treatments. Other versions are in the final phases of clinical testing and should be available within the next year (see list below).

The differences among all these neurotoxins are slight, but they may have an impact depending on your treatment goals. For instance, it may take up to a week for the full effects of Botox to kick in, whereas Dysport may take effect slightly earlier and may spread or migrate from the injection site a touch more. I use both in my practice for different reasons. There are many variables to an individual patient's wants and needs, and I make sure to have as many options on hand as possible.

THE ALTERNATIVES

Here is a complete list of the new and improved toxins of the future to ask about the next time you see your dermatologist:

- Xeomin—Just completed Phase III clinical trials in the United States and is expected to hit the market some time in 2011.

- PurTox—Currently in Phase III clinical trials and also expected to land some time in 2011.

- Lantox—Available only in Asia, Russia, and South America. Be patient. It will come to the United States soon.

- Neuronox—Available in Korea since 2006 and Japan since 2009, it was favorably evaluated against Botox by researchers at Wake Forest University School of Medicine.

- ReVance—A topical version of Botox from California, which will be available for use only at the doctor's office, is in Phase III clinical testing.

- Myoscience—A freezing probe that produces a Botox-like effect.

I have yet to test all these products in my own practice, but the word is that these advancements on Botox are longer lasting with fewer side effects. Consumer demand has created a provider boom, and patients will benefit. Competition is a good thing for your wrinkles as well as for your wallet, since these alternative solutions will gradually force prices down.

There is another potential alternative to temporarily paralyze the facial muscles, and it is not a neurotoxin at all. GFX (glabellar furrow relaxation) is a radiofrequency procedure that lasts approximately 1 year or more. The process causes ablation of the nerves responsible for muscular contraction of the region between the eyebrows. But GFX has not yet been FDA approved and is still in development, so stay tuned!

EXPRESS YOURSELF

When it comes to Botox or other neurotoxins, less is more. Because it's often used excessively these days, the Botox look gets derided, and rightly so. Many patients get so used to being wrinkle-free that they ask for more and more injections and end up having no expression at all. One advantage (which can also be a disadvantage) is that regular use of Botox can have a cumulative effect over time. This may mean continual improvement for some, but others may find their faces becoming more like creepy frozen masks. That's not what Botox is for. It should be used to preserve and improve upon the face you already have naturally, not turn it into something perfectly inhuman.

When applied correctly, Botox creates a subtly refreshed appearance on the forehead, around the eyes, and even around the lower third of the face.

If this is what you are seeking, make sure you find a practitioner with a level of artistic mastery who understands the anatomy of the face. Each muscle has its own weight and strength. A man usually has stronger muscles in the fore-head and between the eyes than a woman, for example, and therefore requires higher dosages of the neurotoxin. Also, there are many variables within an individual face, which is often asymmetrical and requires different amounts of serum on each side.

It bears repeating that the key to a successful Botox treatment is finding a doctor who injects regularly. It is also important to articulate your exact goals when you consult with your physician. For example, if you are seeking treat-ment to open up your eyes and look less tired, or if you want to be able to raise your brows, be specific. I always advise my patients to seek a more natural look and retain some animation in their faces, even if that means a few fine lines.

The areas of the face that have the most repetitive muscle contraction, around the eyes and forehead, respond best to Botox treatment. Frowning can cause deep vertical grooves between the eyebrows that make you look angry. When you take those away, the softening effect of the face is dra-matic. This really is a quick fix. And for the squinters among us, crow's-feet can vanish altogether with a Botox treatment.

Keep in mind that your physician has to customize each treatment and ask how much movement you would like to retain in your face. This is not a cook-book recipe. Each dosage is different depending on what you would like to achieve. You may need less toxin on the upper part of the face, for example, where there is less of a gravity drag and the muscles are weaker. If you want to sculpt a moon face and eliminate "chipmunk cheeks," a popular use for Botox in Asia, the right amount in the right location can have a subtle but significant effect. You can also use these toxins to smooth out frown lines in the lower third of the face or tighten the jawline for a "Nefertiti Lift," a common prac-tice in Europe that is just starting to catch on here. The effect is subtle, but if you're starting to see a little sagging around the jawline, this lift can help.

One of my patients, Alison, was all set to have a surgical face-lift. She was young, in her early forties, and she had one of those soft, full faces that are prone to jowls later in life. Any laxity—a term we dermatologists use to refer to a loss of elasticity—she did have was barely noticeable because Alison took great care of her skin. But her soft jawline was bothersome to her. Alison worked in the fashion industry, where the pressure was on to look flawless, and many of her peers had had mini-face-lifts by the time they hit 40. I wanted to prove to her that there were other options besides surgery. I knew she wouldn't have the patience to wait 6 months for a Thermage treatment to tighten her face, so I suggested she give the Nefertiti Lift a try. Alison was skeptical, but after a few days it produced a slight tightening effect that made all the difference. Botox made her see these nonsurgical options in a different light. Now she's putting off the surgery and is even willing to consider Thermage for her jawline once the Botox wears off.

Though Botox actually takes a lot of skill to administer correctly, some people with no medical background think injecting it is easy and are tempted by the practically instant results. This has led to a lot of overuse and abuse in unqualified hands. Either injecting too close to the upper eyelid or using the wrong dosage altogether creates the common side effects of drooping eyes and heavy eyebrows you may have seen on unfortunate victims who look permanently half-asleep or angry.

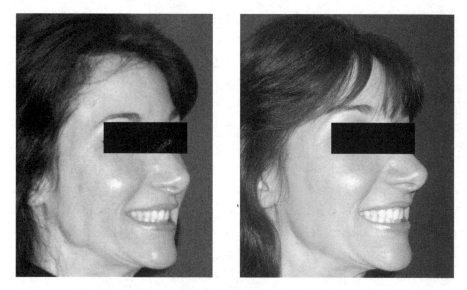

The Nefertiti Lift visibly tightened this patient's jawline.

THE SAFE POISON

On the flip side, the word *toxin* scares a lot of people away from Botox. Though there have been one or two cases of severe side effects over the years from a black market toxin not made by the manufacturers of Botox, there have been *no* reported severe side effects in the United States resulting from Botox manufactured by Allergan. Nevertheless, the FDA required the company to put a black box warning on the label, which makes it necessary for patients to sign a consent form prior to its use. Don't worry, however. In aesthetic medicine, this is a pointless precaution. The quantity of toxin contained in Botox injections for facial use is minimal compared with treatment protocols for musculoskeletal disorders.

As always, common sense should prevail. If you are pregnant or nursing, or if you have a neuromuscular disorder of any kind, you should not use a neurotoxin, period. If you have an infection near the injection site, wait until it clears up. You must also tell your doctor what other medications you are using to avoid any adverse reactions from contraindications. Antibiotics, anti-inflammatories, and even aspirin can cause more bleeding and bruising around the injection site. The same goes for certain herbs or nutritional supplements like St. John's Wort. These rules apply to any injectable treatment.

My patients rarely experience problems with Botox. The procedure itself is virtually painless and takes only a few minutes. The needle is tiny, and you don't even need a numbing cream. I ask my patients to squint and move their faces into certain expressions so I can see exactly where the muscle is, or will be, causing the creases. A few small injections usually take care of the problem areas.

If anything, a few of my more conservative patients come back asking for more. They love their line-free faces, and they want to see how much more Botox can do for them. In certain rare cases, people develop a resistance, or immunity, to Botox after the first couple of treatments. Again, this is not a common problem. But be wary of any doctor who persists in treatment without considering this as a possibility.

Other mostly rare but possible complications from Botox include the following:

- Eyelid droop

- Headache

- Nausea

- Infection and/or swelling around the injection site

- Pain, tenderness, and/or numbness around the injection site

- Redness, bleeding, and/or bruising around the injection site

But most of these complications are not serious, and they are temporary. Good communication with a doctor experienced in using neurotoxins will eliminate most, if not all, of these risks. In a given year, more than 1.5 million patients use Botox for cosmetic purposes, and there has not been one serious incident. Most side effects are purely cosmetic, albeit embarrassing, and usually wear off in a few weeks. That's a better safety rate than aspirin. The numbers don't lie.

CHAPTER EIGHT

HEAL THYSELF

USE WHAT YOU'VE GOT AND PUT THOSE CELLS BACK TO WORK FOR YOU

Imagine you go to your dermatologist's office and he or she draws out a small vial of blood or fat, then spins it in a centrifuge, giving all the growth factors and nutrients that occur naturally in your own cells a great big booster shot. Then that turbocharged mixture is injected back into your body, where it goes to work thickening and plumping your skin exactly where it's needed. The result: elasticity, volume, and that dewy, youthful glow that you thought you'd lost forever. All from your own resources. No other substances. No fillers. *Your* cells and no one else's.

That's not just the future of anti-aging science. It's already here. Cell therapy—the practice of using stem cells and other nutrient-rich biomaterials—has been around for a few years, particularly for use in reconstructive surgery and in helping skin graft patients heal. Healthy cells are taken from undamaged skin and put into a culture to grow new sheets of skin tissue that can be used for grafts. It's far more effective and much less traumatic than traditional skin grafts because patients often reject skin from donor tissue. Stem cell technology can also be used to regenerate bone, cartilage, and hair (more on hair in Chapter 14). It can even be used in breast augmentation as an alternative to implants.

Stem cell therapy goes to the very heart of modern medicine, and it could become the holy grail of anti-aging. These cells know automatically what to repair and where, and they have the unique ability to regenerate and maintain the skin tissue in which they reside. They are a modern-day medical miracle.

But only recently have scientists begun to use this rich body of knowledge in aesthetic medicine. Now widely practiced in Europe and Asia, cell therapy is going to be the next big thing in the United States. Studies to prove the efficacy and longevity of cell therapy are already under way, and it's one of the most promising developments in the field of dermatology. Stem cells are essential to healthy, youthful skin. Studies have shown that aging and damage from UV rays and pollution cause a decrease in stem cell production, with a 29 percent loss in wrinkled areas. Imagine what it could do for our skin if we could replace those lost stem cells. This is an area of age prevention and reversal that's rich in possibilities. I'm investigating various forms of it at my own research center, and other leading dermatologists are already separating fat stem cells from patients' own fat tissue and using their collagen- and tissue-stimulating abilities to enhance the effects of traditional fat transfers and fillers.

There are three emerging cell therapies that use bioactive materials rich in growth factors. One, developed by a company called Isolagen, involves taking a small sample of skin from behind a patient's ear, sending it to a lab to culture the actively producing collagen cells, then reinjecting the substance as filler wherever the patient needs it. This process gives you a potentially unlimited number of fibroblasts, the cells that secrete collagen proteins and help strengthen the connective tissue of the skin. Whether or not this therapy will catch on remains to be seen, however. Sending out samples to be processed over several days is an impractical extra step that may impede its commercial development.

Two other cell therapies that are more likely to take off involve platelet-rich plasma, the use of fat stem cells. I'll explain what they are in a moment, but first I want to make something absolutely clear: In no way, shape, or form has any life been lost in the use or development of these therapies. None of these treatments are using human embryos. In aesthetic medicine, we use either adult stem cells, usually the patient's own, or biomaterials cultured from neonatal foreskins supplied by stem cell banks. There's a lot of baggage associated with the term *stem cells,* and that's a shame. Lives are being saved through stem cell technology every day. Scientists have discovered how to culture human tissue outside the body to be used as skin grafts for bedridden patients recovering from burn wounds and diabetic ulcers. We've only just begun to harness this power to make our lives better in a multitude of ways.

Let me back up a bit by saying that it's still too early to request these treatments along with your annual Botox maintenance, at least here in the United States. The devices that process these cells are still subject to clearance by the FDA—something that should happen any day now. Personally, I am still waiting to test out some of these methods in my own practice. I'm not concerned about safety. Reinjecting biomaterials from your own body is deemed medically safe by the FDA—the body never rejects its own cells—and therefore does not require clinical testing. But as promising as these treatments may be, evidence of their longevity and efficacy is still inconclusive.

It's a catch-22. Because the FDA doesn't require testing, commercial developers don't have the same incentive to invest in all those costly double-blind studies on cell therapies. I'd like to see more controlled testing comparing these injections with traditional fillers like Sculptra and Restylane. Instead we have impressive anecdotal information, but that is all. Be wary of any doctor who pushes these therapies too hard as the next magic bullet. We're not there yet. Also be cynical of any beauty company that touts them in their products. Some topical treatments (which I will discuss) involve stem cells, but be skeptical of beauty companies jumping on the bandwagon. How these formulations work with stem cells isn't as simple and magical as the marketers would have you believe, and only certain products are legitimate. Suffice it to say I'm excited, but not breathless. For now it's better to keep an open mind and consider these therapies along with other, proven methods of building volume, like fillers.

That said, the advent of cell therapies is fantastic news for patients who are averse to using anything but the most natural treatments. On their own, the effects are subtle, but if early results prove consistent, these biomaterials have the potential to greatly prolong and augment existing anti-aging treatments.

VAMPIRE FILLERS

One of the emerging therapies that you're most likely to hear about in beauty magazines in the very near future is platelet-rich plasma (PRP), otherwise known as vampire fillers.

PRP is already widely used by some of Europe's most reputable skin doctors. It does not involve stem cells, but it may be the next best thing. The procedure involves drawing vials of blood from the patient that are then spun down to extract the platelet-rich plasma, a watery substance that's a huge reservoir of bioactive proteins, including growth factors that are vital in the initiation of tissue repair and regeneration. The entire process takes less than 15 minutes and increases the concentration of platelets and growth factors up to 500 percent.

Once this cocktail of nutrients has been harvested and processed, it is strategically injected back into areas of the face that need it most, much the way filler would be used. Alternatively, it could be used as a form of meso-therapy—the injection of small doses all over the face with microneedles—for an overall improvement to the quality of the skin's surface and texture. The plasma injections contain cytokines, which are biologically active mole-cules made up of proteins and peptides that help ensure the equilibrium and rejuvenation of skin cells. These powerful growth factors lead to the stimula-tion of more collagen and other connective tissue, as well as the blood vessels necessary to nourish the skin. The result is fewer lines and added thickness to the outer layer of the dermis.

A growing number of top dermatologists are using PRP therapy. It's not heavily advertised by big drug companies because there's no huge profit to be made from a patient using his or her own cells. But across the pond in particular, this treatment is being added to other best practice treatments as an option particularly suited to patients who don't want an overly aggressive approach.

One of PRP's leading proponents in Europe is my colleague Dr. Sabine Zenker, a respected dermatologist with a small and successful practice in Munich, Germany. Dr. Zenker makes it a point to keep up with whatever is cutting-edge in our field. She has treated dozens of women with PRP and observed some very promising results. PRP is best used in combination with filler or as an adjunct to skin tightening with a laser. But more often than not, German patients prefer to use it on its own. Subtlety is key to the success of Dr. Zenker's practice. For European women, an overdone face or any evidence of the use of filler is a source of deep embarrassment.

"They don't want an obvious change to be seen," says Dr. Zenker. "Not one millimeter of looking injected. Here in Germany, it's a stigma."

COMPLEXION PERFECTION

Angela, a 54-year-old Audi executive from Bavaria, is a typical patient of Dr. Zenker's. Slim, with high cheekbones and attractive features, Angela has done little in the way of anti-aging interventions over the years other than to invest in name-brand skin creams and some Botox. But she was beginning to feel it was time for something more. Her already narrow face was losing volume in the chin region, and her laugh lines and crow's-feet were becoming more noticeable. Colleagues would tell the vivacious blonde that she was looking glum even when she felt fine. She'd wake up after a sound night's sleep and wonder who that tired-looking person was looking back at her in the mirror. A Canadian transplant to Germany, Angela kept hearing about the latest treatments from her more adventurous sister in Vancouver, British Columbia. None of them wowed her until her sister mentioned PRP. Angela was intrigued. She looked up dermatologists in her area, found Dr. Zenker, and began treatments with her. I spoke with her about 6 months after her first series of treatments, and this is what she told me:

I'd had some bad experiences with Botox. Somehow it makes me retain a lot of water. My face swells when I get too much of it, and I look like I have a pair of golf balls under my eyes. But my doctor was confident I could do without Botox or any other filler. When she explained in more detail what was involved in PRP, it just seemed right for me. I really liked the fact that my own blood cells would be going back into my body and working for me. The idea that I would be able to reactivate my cell growth was what made me decide to do it immediately.

The procedure was virtually painless. After a little numbing cream was applied to my face, the doctor went to work, applying the blood mixture to the parts of my face that she felt needed plumping up most: in the hollows under my cheeks, around the mouth, nose, and upper lip, where fine lines were starting to show, below my eyes, and a little on my forehead. She was like a sculptor, molding my face after injecting the plasma and rubbing it smooth. Bruising was minimal and easily covered up with a little foundation. I was at work the next morning, sitting face-to-face with colleagues, and they were none the wiser.

I was warned it would take at least two more treatments spaced 2 weeks apart before I would see results. But I have to say, it was not that long before I started seeing and feeling a difference. When I washed and moisturized my face a few mornings after the first treatment, the skin felt thicker. It sprang back more quickly when I pinched it. About a month and a half later, I could see people giving me a second glance and telling me how rested I looked. You know how critical other women can be. I could tell they were thinking I looked good, like I'd just come back from the spa. I can't necessarily put a number on how many years this has taken off. You couldn't capture the difference in a photograph. But there was a quality to my skin—a certain glow. Overall, there's a marked improvement in my complexion, as if the cells got a good kick start and they're all working again.

I'll probably go back for more in a few months. I want to keep this plumpness up. I don't want it to fade away. Sooner or later I am going to have to face the fact that I may need more aggressive intervention like fillers, even surgery. But for now, I'm happy. I only wish this had been around for me as an option much earlier. Maybe it would have had a much bigger impact if I'd tried this in my thirties and forties. It could have laid a nice foundation.

I think the next step for Angela will be PRP in combination with a filler like Sculptra. The filling agent can provide a scaffolding to hold the plasma fluids in place and give them an opportunity to work where they're most needed. Otherwise, these rich nutrients or growth factors from the blood might migrate from the locations where they're needed most. The PRP will also help prolong the effects of the filler, so that less will be needed and Angela can continue on her chosen path of subtle and gradual improvements.

Like Angela, more patients in the United States will be able to experience PRP in the very near future. But by then the efficacy of this therapy will be substantiated by extensive clinical data. I am going to be a lead researcher helping to bring this new, exciting, and stimulating approach to our shores and discovering the true potential of this futuristic technology.

FACING THE FAT

Fat stem cells are the newest form of cell therapy and one of the most exciting frontiers of anti-aging. In a procedure similar to that of PRP, a small amount of fat is drawn out of the body, this time via minor liposuction, and the substance is spun in a centrifuge. The main difference is that this liquid contains complete stem cells and therefore has many more growth factors than blood plasma alone.

Its contents also make it more controversial than PRP therapy. In addition to the false assumptions about where these stem cells come from, there's a pervading fear that they can somehow stimulate the overproduction of cells and lead to cancer. This is not true, and science and clinical testing results prove it. These fat stem cells are your own tissue, which means there's far less potential for any side effects than there might be from traditional substances we use for volumizing agents or fillers such as hyaluronic acid or animal-based collagen. And there's no danger of these stem cells—or

PRP, for that matter—accidentally migrating to other parts of the body to grow other types of tissue, like cartilage or bone. These stem cells would need much stronger signals than the body is capable of giving to morph into something else.

I can't say for certain whether there are any long-term adverse side effects because we are in the early stages of research, but the regenerative possibilities of fat stem cell transfers are immense. They have been used successfully to treat heart disease and aid in breast reconstruction following a lumpectomy. They help heal tissue damaged by radiation and scarred by burns. If they can do that, it stands to reason that fat stem cells can work wonders in cosmetic medicine, which is much less demanding.

Fat stem cell transfers should not be confused with traditional volumizing agents or transfers of your own preexisting fat. Dermatologists have been harvesting fat tissue removed directly from patients for years, using it as natural fillers for the face. The problem with this procedure is that the fat is reabsorbed quickly into the body, and the cosmetic effect isn't long lasting. And the fat globules are thick, so in less nimble hands, traditional fat transfers can look a little puffy and swollen at first. On the other hand (at least in theory), filling with the watery, stem cell–rich substance that's been separated from the fat tissue should last considerably longer. Patients won't need as much, and stem cells will help produce more volumizing collagen and fat. The bioactive molecules of the fat stem cells will continue to stimulate blood vessel growth, fibroblast cells (the connective tissue that produces collagen), and all the other elements of healthy skin tissue.

Again, it's still too early to tell if fat stem cell fillers will outlast volumizing agents like Sculptra or Radiesse, which I will discuss in Chapter 13. But if the techniques become more advanced, we are going to move more in this direction. The body has a greater tolerance for its native cells, so there are fewer side effects than with many of the fillers we have on the market today.

Again, like PRP, fat stem cells could be used in combination with volumizing filler to help create even more thickness and stimulate collagen. The filler would build a framework within which the cells could regenerate more easily. Patients who've tried this have seen significant increases in elasticity where skin was once slack. Early evidence suggests that stem cells used in this way have also proven effective in softening deep lines, scars, and other defects.

SURFACE SOLUTIONS

There is a lot of confusion out there in the stem cell arena, so let me be clear: Live adult stem cells cannot survive in a jar of skin cream. Rejuvenating stem cell therapy has to be administered by injection in a doctor's office, not smeared onto the skin's surface. However, some topical treatments already on the market (or about to be) mimic stem cells and their components. These compounds can help to fill in fine lines and have been effective in protecting existing stem cells and boosting anti-aging growth factors. Look for products with specialized peptides and epidermal growth factors, which increase the production of fibroblasts.

Christian Dior's Capture XP range uses nutrients found in cell membranes that act as messenger molecules, traveling from cell to cell, improving and protecting tissue that's been damaged by free radicals. It targets and modulates stem cells, keeping them alive for a longer period of time. It does not create additional cells but has a significant ability to protect existing ones from damage and deterioration. In a recent study, lab tests showed that more stem cells were alive in the areas of the skin where the cream was applied, so isolating and treating existing stem cells seems to be the right approach to maintain and prolong healthy, youthful skin. It's an effective topical solution to use in combination with other treatments, but it doesn't go far down beneath the skin's surface, where cell regeneration is needed most. It helps with wrinkling, not sagging.

Another promising topical treatment uses newborn dermal fibroblast cells derived from neonatal foreskins. The cells are grown on beads in controlled bioreactors to maintain an embryonic-like environment with low oxygen and gravity. These conditions basically trick them into thinking they are embryonic stem cells. During this process, the cultured cells secrete a large number of growth factors, including proteins like collagens, laminin, and decorin, which are associated with skin renewal and scar-free healing.

The resulting product is a complex made up of naturally produced cell-signaling molecules and embryonic-like proteins that support the epidermal stem cells that renew skin throughout a lifetime. It's a potent mixture that could drastically reduce the downtime for dermatological procedures such as laser resurfacing. You'll be hearing much more about this new generation of cosmeceuticals in the near future.

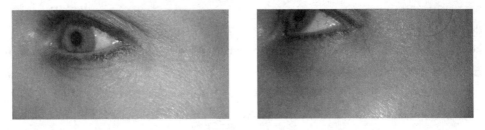

Fine lines around this patient's eyes virtually disappeared after 8 weeks' use of Dior Capture XP.

SMART CELLS

Dr. Gail Naughton, PhD, is one of the lead developers behind many of these emerging treatments. Dr. Naughton got into stem cell technology for aesthetic medicine through her pioneering work producing skin and organ tissue outside the human body. Her research in bioengineering led to new skin-grafting treatments for second- and third-degree burn victims and patients suffering from diabetic foot ulcers, significantly reducing the number of amputations nationwide.

Today, Dr. Naughton is redefining regenerative medicine by manipulating embryonic-like proteins and growth factors taken from infant foreskins to work like stem cells in reproducing healthy skin tissue, cartilage, nails, and hair, meaning patients will be able to get back what they lost under the power of their own cells in ways far beyond the plumping effects of fillers.

Natural enhancement of facial features using biomaterial grafted from your own cells, skin grafts cultured from your own tissue to replace skin lost or damaged following treatment for skin cancer—these could all become accessible to the average patient in just a few years. The building blocks for total rejuvenation will come straight from your own DNA.

CHAPTER NINE

THE FIRST FEATURES TO GO

BAGS, SAGS, AND WRINKLES

It is one of life's raw deals that the two most visible and expressive parts of our face are also among the first to show signs of wear and tear: our eyes and our lips. If there is one feature that my aging patients are most unhappy about, it's their eyes. The eyes are especially vulnerable to the effects of environmental stress and repetitive muscle movement. This is where the skin on our face is thinnest, and it just so happens that the protective oils of the sebaceous glands do not reach the undereye area. So with all our squinting, smiling, and scowling, the dry, fragile skin around our eyes gets plenty of use. No wonder many of us start to see crow's-feet as early as our twenties.

When we're trying to guess someone's true age, the eyes are where we look first, because somewhere along the aging timeline, concealer and a good night's sleep aren't enough to cover up the damage. The skin at the temples gets thin and wrinkly when photoaging runs amok. The tear troughs deepen and darken, making us look tired even when we're not. The upper lids start to droop, eventually falling down to the lash line. Excess skin pigment darkens the lower lids, and feathery lines start to fan the outer corners.

Until recently, the prevailing wisdom was that plastic surgery, the snipping of the upper and lower lids known as an eye job, was the only option. Not so anymore.

Here's the story of one patient who was ready to book an eye job with a plastic surgeon until I persuaded her that she could avoid the knife altogether:

I've had bags under my eyes since I was 3 years old, but it was getting to the point where it was no longer cute. My eyes are deep-set and large, and all it took was a bad night's sleep or a quick cry over a sad movie to turn my little pouches into outright potato sacks. But the tipping point was when my eccentric English uncle came to visit and his first remark upon seeing me was, "Darling, don't you think it's about time you considered an eye job?"

Ouch. That was a bit too honest. But Uncle Tim was right. It wasn't just the extra luggage parked beneath the windows to my soul. My upper lids were starting to droop like an old pair of velvet curtains. You could no longer see the crease between my eyelids, and I was starting to develop a slight hood at the outer corners of my eyes. This was a definite sign of approaching middle age. People were starting to ask me if I was tired when I felt perfectly perky and awake. It was time to do something, and I figured an eye job was my only option. The problem was my fear of the surgery. The idea of having a scalpel anywhere near my eyes made me shudder. What if something went wrong? What if the surgeon cut too much and made me look freakishly wide-eyed? Your eyes are the most memorable feature on your face, and a bad eye job is not a good way to be remembered.

I met with Dr. Sadick to ask him what my options were besides surgery. Through another doctor, I'd had my own fat injected near the top of my cheekbones, a procedure that freshened me up somewhat. But the effects didn't last. Then I tried Restylane with that same doctor, which left me with a bruise under my right eye that lasted for weeks. When it finally healed, I had a bluish tint in the hollow of my eye that never quite went away, so I wasn't particularly sold on fillers. But Dr. Sadick assured me that either Sculptra or my own fat stem cells injected under the muscle close to my orbital bone would smooth out my tear troughs and help my eye bags all but disappear. For my upper lids and brows, he recommended a treatment of Thermage—radiofrequency energy that heats the skin at the dermis level and injures it to help produce collagen. He told me that, conservatively, I could expect perhaps a 30 percent improvement but that these incremental fixes would add to a brighter, more rested look.

A week before my Thermage procedure, I was treated with Dysport (similar to Botox) around my brows to give me a slight arch. I have no wrinkles, at least not yet, but for prevention's sake he threw in a shot between my eyes to stop me from furrowing my brows. I definitely noticed an improvement. The Thermage treatment felt more weird than painful. He put numbing drops in my eyes and inserted a pair of black, ill-fitting contacts to protect my eyeballs from bright lights and the pressure from the handheld tip that would be conducting the energy. The contacts and the feeling they gave me of being totally blind were more irksome than the procedure itself. There were a few moments when the device came near my lash line and it felt as if I'd come into contact with a hot iron, but the whole procedure was over with quickly and the resulting lift was immediately noticeable. I could already see at least a millimeter more of eyelid, and the improvement continued over time. The following week, I came in for the first of a series of deep injections around my lower eyes. Dr. Sadick extracted some fat from my derriere (there was plenty to spare), spun it down in a centrifuge, and prepared the needles. Again, not pleasant, and I was bruised for more than a week after. It took a few months for the total effect of the Thermage and Sculptra treatments to kick in, and the improvement was gradual and subtle, but by the time I returned my uncle's visit, I'd turned back the clock by at least 5 years. I'd say the overall improvement to my upper lids was more like 60 percent, and the lower lids were as smooth and crease-free as they were in my early thirties. It was more than I'd ever hoped for.

"Darling you look fabulous! Now tell me, who did your eye job? I want one, too!"

That, in a nutshell, is a nonsurgical eye-lift. Treatments vary according to the patient's areas of concern, and it takes about 6 months for all the procedures to settle in. And yes, there's some annual maintenance involved. But the overall effect is completely natural and can take away years and either delay or (hopefully) eliminate the need for a surgical eye job.

THE EYES HAVE IT

When it comes to eye-lift surgery, once you start cutting, there's no going back. One surgery isn't going to last you a lifetime, so a decade later you may have to snip away more skin on your upper and lower lids, and the effects will be far from subtle. The skin will become more thin and stretched. In some cases, so much skin is pulled that the inner rim of the eye starts to turn outward. Not attractive and certainly not natural.

With so many alternatives to restoring youth to your eyes, why take that risk? One false move, no matter how small, could have a dramatic impact on the natural you.

Protect those peepers. And don't expect any miracles from an expensive jar of eye cream. Sure, some products help to keep the area moist and protected, but beauty companies know that the eyes are a major area of concern for most women, and even the best make wildly misleading promises. If you do go for an eye cream, look for one that penetrates well and keeps the area under your eyes well moisturized. Generally, a good brand will use the same ingredients that are in the top cosmeceutical creams and serums for the rest of the face, but in lighter formulations, because the skin around the eyes is much more sensitive and products can get in the eyes and irritate them. It's hard to find eye creams with an SPF for this very reason. But they do exist and can help prevent photoaging around your eyes and protect your vision. You can also mix a little sun protection into your regular eye cream, or if that's too irritating, find a good pair of sunglasses with full UV protection.

What eye creams won't do effectively is reverse the damage that's already there. The best you can hope for is to temporarily reduce puffiness, and if the eye cream contains copper peptides or hydroquinone, you might observe a little lightening of pigment and dark circles. There's often some menthol in these products to create a pleasant, cooling sensation and make you think they're actually doing something. But don't be fooled. What you really need under your eyes to combat that tired look is volume, volume, and more volume. And that is not something you can get from a topical. You need filler.

CHARACTER, WITHOUT THE LINES

I like using a patient's own fat under the eye, because it's soft and pliant and gives natural-looking results that are not overfilled. But it's not always practical, because fat needs to be extracted from another part of the body through liposuction, and once you've gone to all that trouble, the effect is not long lasting. Fat fillers can dissipate in as little as 3 months. I usually recommend using Sculptra, one of my favorite volumizing agents, to even out the fat pads under the eyes and eliminate those tear trough grooves (more about Sculptra and other fillers in Chapter 13). The nice thing about Sculptra is that it's longer lasting than most other fillers on the market (up to 2 years versus 6 months to a year) and has the added benefit of helping skin stimulate its own collagen. The injectable poly-L-lactic acid in Sculptra gradually thickens skin and is biocompatible with the body. Also, the viscosity of the substance makes it perfect for the delicate area under the skin. I can inject

Sculptra under the muscle and closer to the orbital bone, then sculpt the volumizing agent for a perfectly smooth look that fills out the lines and creases below the eye.

A moderately ablative laser treatment under the eye like SmartXide or Fraxel will also erase fine lines, get rid of dark circles, and help smooth out the pouches (more about lasers in Chapter 11).

The upper lids tend to fall later in life, and the sooner you do something about it, the less likely you are to need surgery down the road. A little strategically placed Botox, for example, can arch your brows and give the upper lids a slight lift. Tissue-tightening technology also works wonders on the upper lids, opening up the eye without the risk that surgery holds of cutting too much skin. If you do go the plastic surgery route, you are not necessarily finding a permanent solution to the problem of aging eyes, and the more skin you have to cut in future procedures, the more unnatural the look will be.

The tightening effects of these nonsurgical therapies I've mentioned are subtle. But if you start before the problem goes too far, and continue treatments every 1 to 2 years, you will be able to maintain that bright, wide-awake look well into your sixties. Regular shots of Botox in between will also help erase crow's-feet and prevent more lines from forming.

LASHES RX

There is one final thing you can do to take care of your eyes, and it's all in the lashes. Dark, full eye lashes are a classic marker of youth, and they tend to get sparse and fade in color as we age. But flip through any fashion magazine and you'll see models with lush lashes that seem to go on forever. How can ordinary women get the same beguiling look? Well, there are always reusable false eyelashes, layers of thick mascara, or a trip to the salon for individual lash extensions. But these are temporary solutions that may come with some risk. False lashes can cause allergic reactions and eye infections from reusing the same strips, which can collect and accumulate dust and germs. We have also helped patients at my clinic who come in because they have cut their own lashes in an effort to make the false lashes look better. Patients ask us if natural lashes grow back after they've been plucked or cut. Sometimes they do—and sometimes they don't.

The good news is that long lashes are becoming really simple and painless to maintain with the help of a new treatment. In December 2008, Allergan, the company behind Botox, announced FDA approval for Latisse, a new treatment for growing longer, fuller lashes. The drug was originally developed to treat glaucoma, but the developers noticed lush lashes were a side effect, so they decided to market the same formula for aesthetic use. Some experts are worried about Latisse's other possible side effects of red, itchy eyes and changes in eye pigmentation (especially on lighter eyes), but I haven't seen a high incidence of these side effects among my patients, who are overjoyed with their luxurious new lashes and relieved to give up their dependence on more temporary eyelash solutions.

Again, these incremental, youth-enhancing changes are like detailing a car: Each small step needs to be taken to achieve a revitalized look and keep you looking recognizable as *you*. The earlier and more gently you start, the better your chances of looking natural. The same applies to another important feature on your face—your lips. Overdoing cosmetic correction and enhancement of your lips can throw your whole face off balance. I have seen it time and time again. But there are ways to perfect your pout without landing a pair of trout lips.

LIP SYNCHED

I understand the desire to augment lips. A classic marker of aging is the loss of volume in the lips. But when it comes to the mouth, the laugh lines, and the nasolabial folds, overcorrection can look absurd. I have already stated my bias against the sausage lips you see on so many misguided starlets and socialites. They want Angelina Jolie's full, sensuous lips. But Ms. Jolie was born with those lips, so their size and breadth, however full, are in perfect proportion to her face. This is not the case with the thousands of women who are trying too hard to look like her and end up with a distorted and rubbery pout.

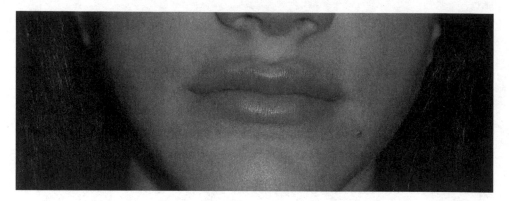

In this case, filler was used above the vermillion border to result in overfilled lips.

When a female patient comes to me to have her lips done, I usually manage to dissuade her from that obvious bee-stung look, and we come up with a conservative plan to achieve truly beautiful, natural-looking lips. It is a multipronged approach that restores youth and enhances what your lips were to begin with.

Instead of focusing on volume and plumping up the lips, address each problem where it occurs and exercise restraint. Start with the lip line, where the first signs of lip aging occur. Otherwise known as the vermilion border, where wet meets dry, tiny channels get carved out by what we call vertical rhytids, or lines. These are barely perceptible at first, but they deepen over time. It's why lipstick starts to feather. The problem is particularly pronounced on smokers, because all that puckering takes its toll. If the lines are very deep, I recommend laser resurfacing. But finer lines can be corrected with tiny amounts of collagen filler right along the border of the mouth, injected laterally using a threading technique to ensure a continuous flow and then massaged in to ensure even distribution and avoid lumps or nodules.

Other small corrections can also rejuvenate the mouth without inflating the lips themselves. A little filler injected into the nasolabial folds can freshen up the whole mouth. Many of my patients also complain of lip droop,

CHAPPED LIP TIPS

While Americans spend a lot of time (and money) protecting their overall skin, they often overlook one crucial part of the face—their lips. The skin on the lips is very thin and fragile, which is why it is critical to care for them on a regular basis. Here are some things you can do before a trip to the dermatologist's office becomes necessary.

THE PROBLEM: CRACKED AND PEELING LIPS

Your lips are exposed to extreme temperatures, sun, and wind, all of which cause moisture loss (whether you are walking outside in the summer or winter, sunbathing, waterskiing, snowboarding, or ice-skating). Cracked lips are a common complaint of people who live in dry and humid weather conditions or spend many hours in centrally heated or air-conditioned rooms.

THE TREATMENT

Refrain from the common reaction of licking your lips, which can be drying. Instead, help them retain their natural moisture by using a quality lip balm with an SPF if possible. Great products include Clinique Superbalm, Labello, and Neutrogena Lip Moisturizer. Exfoliate lips on a regular basis just as you would the rest of your face, using Smashbox Emulsion Lip Exfoliant or Philosophy Kiss Me Exfoliating Lip Scrub. A little sugar and olive oil also does the trick.

when the corners of their mouths turn down and form tiny lines that extend outward. This is easily corrected with a small quantity of filler injected at the corners or even a tiny amount of Botox or Dysport to lift the area and prevent further lines.

Again, be conservative. Overcorrection can erase the philtrum, the midline grove between your nostril and mouth that creates your pout or "Cupid's bow." A philtrum is a nice thing to hold on to if you'd prefer not to look like a monkey. If you are at all concerned about this and other problems resulting from excess augmentation, you may want to try correcting your lips with something reversible at first, like a hyaluronic acid–based filler. Keep in mind that the top lip should always be thinner than the bottom lip.

Whatever you do to your lips, don't let anyone talk you into permanent fillers, because you will live to regret it. I won't name names, but you may recognize a few actresses who opted for silicone, even though this implant has not been FDA approved for use in the lips. Silicone can cause scarring, lumps, and bumps, and because it does not age with your lips, your skin could drape around atrophied silicone and create distortions that can be only partially corrected through surgical excision. Semipermanent fillers with a harder texture, like Radiesse, are also a bad idea for the lips because of the greater chance for lumps, bumps, and distortions.

Throughout this book, I have often repeated the "less is more" maxim, and it is especially true when it comes to your eyes and your lips. Both are key facets of your natural beauty, so I implore you to treasure what you already have and stick to subtle improvements.

CHAPTER TEN

THE FLAWS TO FOLLOW

YOU DON'T HAVE TO GO THROUGH LIFE WEARING GLOVES OR A TURTLENECK

Many of my patients approach age reversal as though they are on a serious mission. They start with their faces, correcting all those tiny flaws and markers of aging that show up first on the eyes, forehead, and lips, then slowly make their way down their bodies: taking care of sagging necks and jawlines, ropy hands, droopy knees, and dimpled legs. Increasingly, women (and some men) are requesting procedures in the most unexpected places. They've done everything right in the face, where most people look first, but in today's judgmental world, not even the elbows are safe from scrutiny. My patients want it all. And they can have it all.

Unless you are blessed with a lantern jaw and a swan neck, the area from the jawline to the chest is usually the next part of the body after the face to betray our age. We don't necessarily think of it first, but the loss of firmness in the neck tends to pull everything down, and it can happen as early as our mid-thirties. Depending on the shape of your face and where you tend to gain weight, that pocket of skin right below the chin can lose elasticity and droop in a way that adds years to your profile. Most people automatically assume that the only way to correct this is with a mini-face-lift—cutting the skin behind the ears and pulling back the excess. But surgery is neither your only nor your best option. Let me share the story of my co-writer, Samantha, who hated her neck to the point where she wouldn't even allow her picture to be taken in profile. Sam decided to do something about it but avoid going under the knife:

I was kicking myself that I hadn't researched my options more when I first heard about laser-assisted lipo from Dr. Sadick. I'd always hated my neck, which was getting progressively flabbier with age, so a few months earlier I'd had a traditional neck lipo procedure with another doctor—my first experience with any kind of cosmetic procedure. The operation was successful. Recovery was painful and the downtime was inconvenient, but my neck was skinnier. I'd made it into that window where my skin still had enough elasticity to bounce back from the loss of volume, so I did not have to take the more drastic step of a neck-lift with cutting and stitches. Still, I wasn't satisfied. It wasn't quite the Audrey Hepburn neck-line I was hoping for. There were those telltale vertical bands of loose skin where the fat used to be, and it bothered me. The skin-tightening effect of a laser fiber under my skin would have produced more collagen and tightened everything up, but I didn't know about the technology at the time. Oh well, I figured. It's too late now. This is the best it can be.

Not so, said Dr. Sadick. Thermage might just do the trick. He didn't promise me a completely smooth neckline, but at least I could expect a 30 to 50 percent improvement in one shot, and that alone would make a big difference. I was skeptical but desperate enough to give it a try.

First, he drew a grid from my jawline, behind my ears, and down to my collarbone, mapping out small squares where the treatment would concentrate its energy. Then he trained the handheld device's tip on the jawbone near my ear and zapped. After a few beeps there was an energy spike that felt like intense heat. It wasn't comfortable. But as he progressed toward the middle of my throat, the intensity of the heat subsided and for the most part it was bearable. It was oddly comforting knowing that the first few minutes would be the worst. I could brace myself. After about 45 minutes the procedure was over and the Percocet was finally kicking in. Better late than never. I expected to see singe marks, but there was only a slight redness that was gone after 20 minutes. I thought I could see a little improvement, although it was probably some initial swelling. Dr. Sadick warned me I'd have to be patient. It takes a few months for the collagen to really go to work.

A few weeks later, the definition to my jawline was more pronounced and things did look a little tighter below my chin. Six months later, my neck looked even better. I'm thrilled with my newly taut jawline and the virtual disappearance of my turkey neck.

A year later, I decided to go for a follow-up treatment. My neck still looked good, but I felt I needed an extra blast for a perfectly taut gorge. I'd heard the new technology was much more comfortable. I was skeptical, and once again I braced myself for that hot-iron sensation. But the process was much less painful and traumatic than my first round. You feel a surge of heat, quickly followed by a cool rush on the site being treated. You rarely, if ever, feel you're going to burn. And on those sensitive spots near the outer jawline and under the ear, where the energy reflects off the bone and magnifies the discomfort, Dr. Sadick buzzed me using a new comfort technology handpiece designed to trick the brain and distract it from the pain. It worked, although it was rarely necessary during the procedure.

The beauty of the upgraded Thermage technology is that it allows the doctor to deliver more intense heat for a greater tightening effect. This time around, I noticed tightening within a month, and it only got

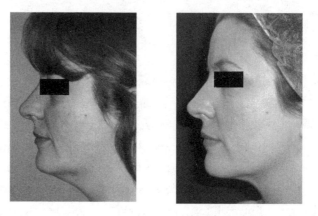

A combination of neck liposuction followed by two Thermage treatments dramatically improved Sam's neckline.

better. It may last 1 year or 2 this time, but I don't dread having to go back for a touch-up. I'm going to keep this up with the annual or biannual treatments, especially knowing how pain-free the procedure is. You could almost call it relaxing. Well, almost.

The best part is that now I mug for every camera shot. I used to avoid those sideways glances in the mirror, but now I catch glimpses of myself in profile and smile. Two years ago, I never would have thought this was possible. I would draw my index finger across my neck to pull back the skin and imagine what it would be like if it was nice and taut. But today I couldn't be more proud of my new neck. Dr. Sadick gave me that movie-star jawline I thought I could never have!

Never underestimate the glory of a taut, youthful neckline. Many of my patients—especially those fortunate enough to have nice firm necks well into middle age—need to be reminded to protect what they have. How many of you actually apply moisturizers and sunscreens to your neck on a daily basis? Be honest. While it's true that a cream isn't going to fix the pull of gravity or the influence of genetics, the skin below the jawline is delicate and it needs all the extra help it can get to maintain good definition and elasticity.

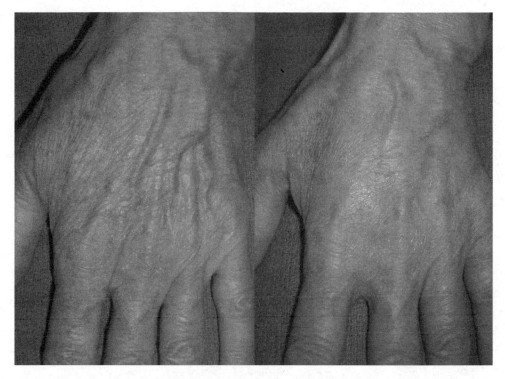

Protruding veins and visible tendons in this patient's hands are dramatically softened with appropriate placement of filler.

HANDS DOWN

There are many other areas that we tend to neglect until we notice the skin is no longer as firm and smooth as it used to be. Once women start looking past their faces and necks, they usually notice their hands. Let's face it—protruding veins and joints, brown spots, and puckered skin on your digits are dead giveaways of aging. As the years add on, our hands lose firmness and plumpness and begin to look bony and fragile, with a thin, papery skin texture that's not sexy.

Combating the aging hand syndrome takes more than hand cream (though that simple step does make a difference, especially when it includes Retin-A). The latest technology has given us a set of procedures that will have effects

ITSY-BITSY SPIDER VEINS

Though the terms *spider veins* and *varicose veins* are often used interchangeably to refer to those unsightly bluish veins that often appear on aging legs, the two conditions are different. Varicose veins are large, bulging veins that are usually found in the legs and feet but can also appear elsewhere on the body, including the hands. In most cases, they are merely inconvenient and cosmetically unappealing, but they can become painful and may indicate underlying circulatory problems. On the other hand, telangiectasias, or spider veins, are not raised or palpable. They are clusters of small red or purple blood vessels that can appear on the thighs, calves, ankles, feet, and occasionally the face. Both conditions are caused by genetic factors and/or poor circulation. Some people are more prone to weak valves in their blood vessels that break down over time, allowing blood to backflow through them. As blood builds up in the lower extremities, pressure increases, resulting in the formation of these veins. Weight gain, pregnancy, hormonal changes, smoking, crossing legs or standing for extended periods, and trauma or impact from running can all exacerbate these conditions, which affect 20 to 41 percent of women and 6 to 15 percent of men in the United States.[8] Women are more prone to varicose veins because they undergo more hormonal fluctuations associated with pregnancy, birth control, menstruation, and menopause.

While not necessarily medically serious, spider and varicose veins are distressing for patients. Many refuse to wear anything that will reveal their extremities and won't expose them on the beach or at the pool. But solutions to the problem are much easier than a traditional phlebectomy—literally the stripping or surgical removal of veins—which is painful and can leave railroad-track scars along the legs. Now we have lasers and injectable agents to get rid of the offending veins. The best treatment for you will depend on the outcome of your diagnostic duplex ultrasound—a painless, non-invasive procedure that uses sound waves to obtain a picture that allows your doctor to see the diameter of the vein as well as the velocity and direction of the blood flow within it. The ultrasound will also rule out any circulatory or underlying medical reasons for the veins. Once you get the all-clear for cosmetic treatment, these are your options:

◆ **Laser Vein Removal**—This procedure can erase spider veins in a flash and, when performed with an endovascular laser treatment, commonly known as EVLT, can also address more problematic varicose veins. During the EVLT, a thin laser fiber is inserted into the vein near the knee and guided through the vessel via ultrasound. The fiber then delivers laser energy to the varicose vein, collapsing it and diverting blood flow to other veins nearby that work properly. The procedure is well tolerated by patients, and 2 years postprocedure, most experience a varicose recurrence rate of less than 7 percent, according to a study recently published by the Sadick Research Group.[9] In short, EVLT is the most effective treatment for those with more pronounced vein problems. With the latest laser technologies, darker skin types can also be treated for leg veins with minimal risk of burning or discoloration of the epidermis.

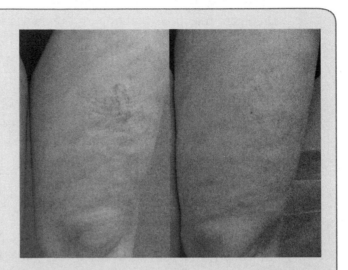

After just two sclerotherapy treatments, this patient shows about a 70% reduction in visible leg veins.

◆ **Sclerotherapy**—This injection vein treatment using a liquid or foam sclerosing agent has long been considered the gold standard in eliminating both spider and varicose veins. The sclerosing agent causes the veins to collapse and close, and they are eventually replaced by scar tissue. The advantage of foam sclerotherapy is that a given concentration of liquid in foam form has greater potency and requires fewer treatment sessions than the traditional liquid form of sclerotherapy. New techniques and sclerosants also enable doctors to treat larger-diameter vessels more effectively. While sclerotherapy treatments certainly work and offer minimal discomfort and downtime, they are more technique dependent than laser vein treatment, so seek an experienced doctor.

◆ **Ambulatory Phlebectomy**—Traditional vein removal surgery may be necessary in cases where varicose veins are too large to be treated with injection removal methods but too small for laser vein treatment. However, there are new microincision techniques that minimize pain, scarring, and downtime, so if you do require an ambulatory phlebectomy, you need not fear the worst.

similar to those we have been able to accomplish for the face. Radiesse or Sculptra injections replump and replenish volume to the backs of the hands to provide a supple and youthful appearance. Placed beneath the skin, these volumizing agents raise the skin level so that tendons, joints, and veins lose their prominence. Laser treatments also help shrink pores and smooth out wrinkles. It's basically a nonsurgical hand-lift. Fractional and Q-switched lasers can also remove pigmented spots and smooth out hand wrinkles (more to come on lasers in Chapter 11).

Foam sclerotherapy—a foamed solution that is injected directly into veins to thicken the blood and cut off the flow to the protruding vessel—is another way to smooth out ropy hands. The endovenous laser, which I pioneered, is also very effective. It's a quick outpatient procedure performed under local anesthetic that uses a tiny laser fiber under the skin to target and seal off the leaky veins that cause protrusions.

One of my patients, Amy, recently opted for this treatment when she got engaged to her much younger boyfriend. Amy had taken great care of her face over the years, coming to me regularly for facial peels, Botox, and fillers, but her future in-laws didn't know her real age, and she didn't particularly want them to know. Not to mention the fact that she didn't want her weathered hands appearing in her wedding photos. Now Amy has a pair of supple, youthful hands to match her beautiful face.

QUICK FIXES

The use of fillers and injectable fat grafts from the neck down is a burgeoning trend in the dermatology field. Done right, a few judicious injections can fill out the divots and dimples caused by cellulite on the thighs or buttocks and correct the adhesions left behind by liposuction procedures. These off-face procedures are not yet widespread and are very technique dependent, but they are certainly a promising new direction in the field that will be driven by consumer demand.

While weight loss may be the ultimate goal for many aging individuals, women tend to lose their feminine curves as they age, and a fair amount come to my practice seeking ways to restore the roundness of their derrieres or to add softness to a bony sternum. Small amounts of volumetric fillers like Sculptra and hyaluronic acid can fill out the space between the breasts where skin gets thin and hollow with age. Some doctors are even experimenting with larger-scale fat grafting, removing fat tissue from thighs or the stomach to inject into the crease where the buttocks meet the top of the leg to give a sagging butt a lift. And new hyaluronic acid–based fillers are being designed to treat much larger areas of the body.

Of course, there is a risk of complications with these techniques, which have not yet proven to be entirely safe or cosmetically effective. Only a handful of practitioners are currently performing them. Fat tends to migrate, and large volumes would be required to produce real body-contouring effects. That degree of fat grafting could also cause infections, and in cases where doctors are experimenting with fat and fat stem cell grafting to breasts—a potentially exciting alternative to breast implants—calcifications and nodules can occur that may interfere with mammogram readings. Nevertheless, fat transfers are the new frontier in body contouring and with further research, testing, and refinement could become an industry standard for perfecting and enhancing the shape of arms, legs, breasts, hips, butts—virtually anywhere a patient would like to see a little extra curve and volume.

THE LAST TO GO

They say the legs are the last to go, and I certainly know plenty of women in their sixties and seventies with gorgeous gams. But there are still problem areas in the limbs that concern patients when they enter their forties and fifties. One famous actress in her mid-forties once told me that if there was one thing she could change about herself, it would be her knees. She was in good shape, but gravity was pulling on the fat and skin above her kneecaps. This lumpy, droopy look to the skin on and around her knees was simply the result of time and the genetic shape of her leg, but she was so self-conscious that she would never go out in public wearing above-the-knee hemlines or shorts.

Fortunately, it was an easy fix. While laser lipolysis—the extraction of laser-heated and liquefied fat—is technically surgical because it involves an incision, that incision is so tiny and the downtime so minimal that it almost doesn't count! Those gnarly knees were gone after the procedure, and after a week in a compression bandage, the skin around them looked firm and toned. Laser lipolysis is also a great tool for other small areas of the body that need a lift. It can add contour to "cankles"—when you can't tell where the calf meets the ankle—and slim down heavy calves. It can also get rid of that pocket of fat at the top of the arms known as bat wings that become stubbornly resistant to weight training as we age (more on the advantages of laser lipolysis in Chapter 15).

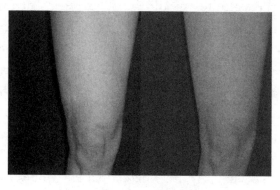

Laser lipolysis was used to generally contour this patient's legs. Note the tightening effect just above the knee.

That said, you don't need even minimally invasive procedures like laser lipolysis to correct most problems below the neckline. Fillers can be used to add definition to slack jawlines and as an alternative to lipolysis to give a lift to drooping kneecaps. Thermage not only has proven effective at tightening turkey necks, but works well with other isolated trouble spots off the face like the arms and knees. And lasers such as Fraxel can attack myriad problems below the face, helping resurface sun-damaged or photoaged skin on the chest. Like hand veins, leg veins can be zapped with light-based lasers (see "Itsy-Bitsy Spider Veins" on page 116 for more on spider and varicose veins). Finally, SmartXide, which is similar to Fraxel but with different wavelengths, can improve laxity in the neck and treat raw, red, and bumpy skin anywhere on the body.

By no means am I encouraging you to scrutinize your body for flaws to correct. Just know that if you are self-conscious about something and want help, you can get it! Whatever may be the next part of your body to go, there is a cutting-edge technology to treat it. No problem lacks a safe and effective nonsurgical solution. Again, nobody can have perfection. But anyone can attain the New Natural.

PART III

REVERSE

(Ages 40 to 80 . . .)

CHAPTER ELEVEN

LASER'S EDGE

YOUR BEST NEW WEAPON AGAINST THE SURGEON'S KNIFE

Accent, SmartXide, Gemini . . . Every time you visit the dermatologist's office, you may notice another pamphlet for a new machine on display, each one harnessing some type of energy to tighten skin, stimulate the growth of collagen, or smooth out wrinkles, all without surgery. This is the future of age prevention and reversal, and the technology can produce dramatic results approaching surgery, albeit in the New Natural way. But not all of these machines were created equal. The trick is to sort out which device will work best for you.

Lasers have come a long way since they were first introduced in dermatologists' offices in the 1970s. Laser is an acronym that stands for light amplification by stimulated emission of radiation. It produces an intense and focused beam of light that can cut, cauterize, or vaporize blood vessels and skin tissue, depending on the intensity, wavelength range, and duration. Lasers can produce specific colors of light that work best on a certain problem.

Green, for example, works well on yellowish and brown areas of pigmentation, like age spots. Blue light performs well on acne. Short pulses of yellow light are more precisely absorbed by hemoglobin, so it works on blood vessel disorders like port wine stains and red nose syndrome. Red light can treat everything from freckles and brown pigment lesions to unwanted hair, even tattoos. It all depends on the speed and strength of the energy and the practitioner's ability to custom-fit each treatment.

Today we have a multitude of light and heat devices that can treat skin conditions with minimal risk of surface injury. It's up to the doctor to select the correct device, adjusted to the safest and most effective settings.

As someone who researches and develops many kinds of laser technology for approval by the FDA, I get to see all that's new and on the horizon in non-ablative and ablative devices that tighten and correct skin and stimulate collagen. From surface problems like excess skin pigment, acne, light scarring, and wrinkles to deeper problems within the dermis such as skin folds and laxity, the technology exists to perfect skin at every level.

There is no question that lasers can do great things—multiple forms of light, radiofrequency, heat, and cold can all interact with human tissue for myriad benefits. Lasers can remove hair and visibly reverse skin damage. They can also dissolve fat as part of a liposuction procedure. In fact, for every marker of aging there is at least one new machine to zap it out of existence. And one type of energy and power level may not be appropriate for everyone. Very wrinkled skin might require a more ablative laser therapy that causes surface injury and involves more downtime for recovery, for example. Ablative refers to the vaporizing power of the laser energy, which blasts away at the outer layers of the epidermis, causing it to blister and then crust over, revealing fresh new skin tissue as it heals. Non-ablative devices, however, leave the skin's surface intact and go to work at the dermis level. A younger patient who wants more taut skin might opt for a non-ablative treatment such as Thermage, for example, which uses radiofrequency energy to heat and tighten skin below the surface.

We've been touching on light lasers and other types of energy throughout this book because they have applications beyond the face—for hair growth, body contouring, and the removal of varicose veins. But in this chapter, I am going to focus on which machines work best to correct skin flaws and reverse the signs of aging from the neck up. This is what they were originally designed to do, and it's still the most common area of interest for patients.

APPROACH WITH CAUTION

Do keep in mind that when placed in the wrong hands, lasers can lead to severe damage. You can liken lasers to heat weapons. If too much energy is applied, skin burns and scarring can result. If you are going in for any type of laser procedure, you want a physician, a licensed physician assistant, a nurse practitioner, or a registered nurse performing it. Also, don't have laser treatments when you are tanned because the laser light is picked up by darker skin pigmentation and you could end up looking discolored and blotchy. Lasers are much less effective at removing unwanted hair or diminishing wrinkles on tanned skin.

If the laser treatment is extremely painful, tell your doctor so he or she can lower the settings. A good physician will want to know your concerns and do everything possible to prevent injury. If after the treatment your skin is persistently red or there is blistering, be sure to go right back to your doctor to be treated with the proper healing and lubricating agents to minimize the chance of scarring. This is an area of aesthetic medicine where the patient needs to be especially vigilant. If something doesn't feel right, speak up. I've seen too many disasters that resulted from practitioners who didn't fully understand how to use this technology.

Despite these risks, laser treatment is the preferred option for my more conservative patients who shun fillers and surgery. The key is to find the appropriate technology to match the condition to be treated. It's all too easy for patients to waste thousands of dollars and see little benefit. That's what gives lasers a bad name. There's also a tendency for manufacturers of this technology, and some of the doctors who just bought the new machines, to overpromise and underdeliver. But when they're used correctly, they can be just as effective as surgery.

NO NEEDLES, NO BLADES

Sarah is a beauty-savvy New York financial executive who really does her research. I was impressed by how much she knew about the latest non-invasive approaches in aesthetic medicine. Laser treatment is what drew her to my practice. As long as no scalpels or needles are involved, Sarah will try whatever skin care technology is considered the most cutting-edge, and now at 36, she's had just about every type of laser resurfacing treatment to correct her acne scars. In her early twenties, she'd developed a bad case of cystic adult acne and her dermatologist at the time prescribed Accutane, a form of vitamin A that dries up the sebaceous glands. The problem was that Accutane is meant only for the severest form of acne after other options fail. Sarah's problem wasn't that severe, and the side effects of the cure were much worse than the condition. She took too much and her skin dried out. As a result of the drying, her skin didn't have the collagen it needed to heal properly, and the acne left behind depressions on the surface that made her very self-conscious.

By the time she got to me, at age 33, Sarah had the skin of a much older woman. It didn't help that the young lady, a pretty blonde of Anglo-Irish descent, had misspent her youth sun worshipping and lying on tanning beds. She went to another doctor before she read about me, and he gave her silicone injections to even out the scars, but they did little to help. Glycolic acid peels—superficial chemical peels that remove the top layer of skin—were not effective, either. Her doctor then recommended Polaris, a non-ablative laser that combines radiofrequency with pulsed light, but she found it extremely painful and the improvements were marginal because Polaris was never meant to treat scarring. It's more for light wrinkling like crow's-feet and frown lines, neither of which was an issue for Sarah. Needless to say, this disappointing experience made Sarah very skeptical about today's skin care technology. After all that time and money spent on procedures, she saw a 10 percent improvement at best.

When she stepped into my office seeking real solutions to her scars, I decided that we should proceed cautiously. Sarah had highly sensitive skin, and she was prone to keloids—the growth of excess scar tissue that's lumpy and often discolored. We started her on Laser Genesis, a non-ablative technology that uses concentrated light at the surface and at a deeper layer of the dermis to trigger collagen production and tighten skin. It also works to get rid of diffuse redness, shrink the pores, and generally smooth out the overall texture of the skin. It takes four to six treatments and is reassuring for beginners because it's gentle, there is little to no downtime, and the risk of injury is minimal. It is also safe for most skin types, and the process is not as painful as with other non-ablative and ablative technologies. Sarah described it as feeling like a burst of heat on her face, without a burning sensation, and once she got used to the procedure she found it therapeutic and relaxing enough to put her to sleep.

The Laser Genesis improved the color and texture of Sarah's skin, but she needed further treatment to truly eliminate her scars. We decided to graduate her to Fraxel, which consists of several strengths and generations that I will detail later in this chapter. In Sarah's case, we used Fraxel re:store, the original application that is the midlevel Fraxel treatment in terms of aggressiveness. Fraxel re:store is ideally suited for resurfacing damaged skin with minimal downtime and is most commonly used for treating moderate surface flaws like acne and surgical scars as well as wrinkles and skin discoloration.

Treatment of acne scars requires the removal of damaged skin and the production of new collagen to improve the area's tone and texture from deep within the dermis, and the Fraxel treatment accomplishes both. Microscopic laser columns penetrate a fraction at a time, leaving surrounding tissue intact so that healing is fast. It literally rebuilds the damaged cells from the inside out. The result is improved elasticity and texture, and because of the precision of the technology, healthy tissue remains intact, with minimal discomfort or downtime.

Since Sarah's past experiences with lasers made her especially cautious, she took it upon herself to thoroughly research the safety and efficacy of the technology, and rightly so. I wish all patients were as circumspect. This was a big commitment in terms of time and money. Fraxel costs between

$750 and $1,500 per session, and Sarah would need at least six sessions spaced a few weeks apart. By contrast, the Laser Genesis is $200 to $400 per session.

Fraxel ended up passing Sarah's inspection, but we started slowly, on the gentlest of the machine's settings. Though the risks of the procedure are low, the last thing we wanted to do was aggravate Sarah's already sensitive and damaged skin.

Sarah reacted well to the treatment. She felt an increased sensation of heat as we passed the laser device over her face, but she told us the 25-minute session was more than tolerable. To minimize discomfort during the procedure, we applied a topical anesthetic and used cold air on the treatment area. Post-procedure, she said it felt as though she had a sunburn, but the sensation diminished after a couple of hours. There was also a little swelling, but that subsided after a day. Over the next week, her skin went from pinkish to bronzed, as if she'd spent too much time in the sun. She moisturized her face and exfoliated when the skin started to peel, a perfectly normal reaction that shows the procedure is working. We advised her to avoid the sun, wear a hat, and apply sunscreen with an SPF of at least 20 every day.

BEST FACE FORWARD

As Sarah's tolerance built, we increased the Fraxel settings. She's now completed her eighth session, and the overall improvement to her skin's texture is about 70 percent compared with when she first stepped into my office. She's already showing more confidence. She used to style her hair so it would cover as much of her face as possible, and now she pulls it back into a ponytail. Her skin looks great: Her pores are invisible, her skin tone is even, and the pockmarks are barely noticeable.

The damage that Accutane and sun worshipping left on Sarah's face was severe, but today you'd never know how rough it once looked. And another happy side effect of all this laser energy has been a noticeable tightening of the skin on her face and neck. She looks closer to 28 than 36.

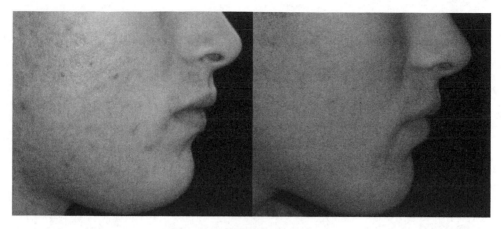

Dramatic improvement of acne scars is visible after 3 Fraxel treatments on this male patient.

"All this time I've spent with lasers will probably mean I'll always look 10 years younger than my actual age," says Sarah. "I can live with that!"

There are laser and other energy treatments that are right for every type of skin problem. But be wary of any doctor who champions only one kind. Sometimes the best solutions require multiple protocols, and it's vital to take into consideration the skin type and pain tolerance of each patient. Here's a breakdown of the latest technology according to strength, treatment, and energy type:

INTENSE PULSED LIGHT (IPL)

IPL, the most popular form of laser treatment for skin, is broadband light delivered in high-intensity pulses. It is one of the mildest treatments for treating uneven skin tone, fine lines, diffuse redness and rosacea, small veins, and enlarged pores. The effect is known as a photofacial, although there are numerous technologies that achieve varying results. It is usually non-ablative, meaning it does not touch or injure the skin's surface. There is virtually no recovery or downtime, just a little redness and swelling. The object of IPL is to deliver as much energy to a site in as short a time as possible to vaporize certain cells and blood vessels for more targeted treatment. The wavelength, power output, and color of a particular laser determine its cosmetic application. When IPL light is directed at skin tissue, its energy is absorbed by water or pigments in the skin. These pigments include hemoglobin, a protein that makes blood red, and melanin, the pigment responsible for tanning and for producing brown spots on the skin, which absorb a broad spectrum of laser light. IPL can be used anywhere around the face, chest, and eyes. Here are a few examples of IPL technology:

- Laser Genesis (by Cutera): Uses microbeams to protect the epidermis. It targets tiny veins, stimulates collagen production, and improves wrinkles with gentle heating. It also corrects diffuse redness and rosacea, smooths skin texture, and shrinks pore size. But this is not the most powerful of the IPL lasers, and it is best used on the more minor skin flaws. It works almost like a light glycolic skin peel. One mode of treatment to give the skin an overall glow before a big event involves holding the wand handpiece far from the face and passing it over the skin's surface to gently kill bacteria in the pores and shrink them. Patients can actually hear a popping sound as the dirt, oil, and bacteria vaporize from the pores, which automatically shrink to give skin a nice smooth texture that lasts for a few weeks.

- StarLux (by Palomar Medical): Offers multiple IPL wavelength settings, including fractional and infrared handpieces. I like their MaxG handpiece for treating pigment. The green light laser produces a wavelength that is highly absorbed by melanin, causing café au lait discolorations common with aging, particularly on the backs of the hands, to all but disappear. The melanin is heated and the damaged pigmented lesion is naturally sloughed off as the skin exfoliates. Similar results are seen in the treatment of vascular lesions. The green light is absorbed particularly well by the redness in the skin, and the resulting thermal action causes the offending blood vessel to degenerate and disappear over two to three treatment sessions of about 20 minutes each.

- LimeLight (by Cutera): Particularly effective for low-contrast pigment. Like the LuxG, it works well on redness and brown spots, and its power can be adjusted easily according to skin color and type. Low-contrast pigmentation is a clinical challenge, and while most IPLs can treat only high-contrast pigmentation, LimeLight can treat both. Three distinct preset programs (520 to 1,100 nanometers) enable the practitioner to customize the treatment for a range of skin types and problems, including advanced rosacea and acne, in one session. There's also a cooling device on the tip of the handpiece to cool the skin before and after each laser pulse. Treatments take about 20 minutes each and are recommended once a month for 3 to 5 months.

- Vbeam (by Candela): A pulsed dye laser that uses long pulses for a gentle heating impact and multiple wavelengths for deep penetration. As with the LuxG, its handpiece delivers a cooling spray of air to the treatment site to reduce the risk of blistering or redness. The laser is set to target the darker, dense blood vessels at deeper layers of the skin that cause red spots, birthmarks, and port wine stains.

- RevLite (by HOYA ConBio): This laser works non-ablatively to correct a wide range of conditions, including wrinkles, discolorations, age spots, pigment lesions, and unwanted tattoos. It works beneath the surface of the skin to stimulate collagen production. As the deeper skin tissues are heated, the skin matrix is remodeled and patients see an improvement in skin texture, tone, wrinkling, and pores. I like RevLite for the computer control it offers, switching between red, green, and yellow beams depending on the problem being treated. It emits short light pulses that resemble the snap of a thin rubber band on the skin. The laser treatment lasts no more than 20 minutes and requires no downtime. It takes up to three treatments spaced a few weeks apart to see complete results.

THE ABLATIVES

Ablative laser treatments—also known as lasabrasion—operate on much more powerful settings than non-ablative lasers, to injure the skin in a safe, controlled way. This action rejuvenates the epidermis and tightens skin as it heals and produces more collagen. A powerful laser beam essentially vaporizes the aged and damaged upper layers of tissue so that newer, healthier

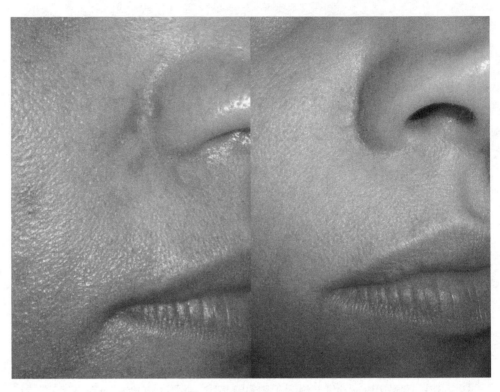

Divots and discoloration around this patient's nose are erased with the use of the RevLite laser.

cells can emerge. Most research studies agree that when performed properly, ablative laser resurfacing can visibly reduce the appearance of fine lines and, in some cases, deep wrinkles, and the effects can last up to 2 years. It is used either on the entire face or just in the areas around the eyes and mouth. Of course, there are injury risks when used improperly, and pain and recovery time vary widely depending on the strength of the treatment. But newer technology minimizes risk by damaging less of the surrounding tissue. Potential adverse reactions include excessive scarring, infection, loss of normal skin pigmentation, skin redness, and dryness. Since people with darker skin are more likely to develop uneven pigmentation, their doctor should perform a patch test prior to treatment to determine whether the treatment will cause discoloration. Generally, this skin tone responds better to the longer wavelengths of 1,064 nanometers. Patients like Sarah, who were on Accutane, as well as those with certain connective tissue disorders, are more susceptible to scarring. Laser peels can also activate the herpes virus or aggravate inflammatory skin conditions. Depending on the patient's medical history, the physician should prescribe and administer an oral antiviral drug and/or antibiotics before and after the procedure. But in the hands of a physician with extensive experience in this type of technology, side effects are relatively rare, and the final result and improvement to skin texture can be dramatic and well worth the temporary discomfort.

Here is a short history of ablative laser options:

• CO_2—Traditional carbon dioxide lasers are perhaps the most aggressive form of resurfacing treatment. This was the first resurfacing laser system,

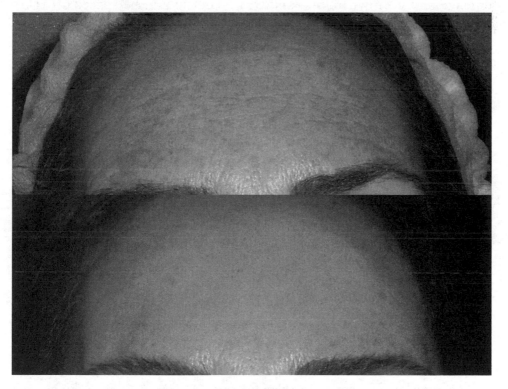

Pigment, tone, texture, and lines on this patient's forehead are dramatically improved using ablative laser technology.

and it is used for treating deep wrinkles and folds, smoothing sun-damaged skin, obliterating the deep vertical wrinkles that occur around an aging mouth, and eradicating deep acne scars. But CO_2 lasers require a longer recovery time than any other type of resurfacing laser technology, and there's a greater risk of complications. Be prepared to look like a burn victim the first several days after treatment. Your skin will ooze before it crusts over. This is a powerful piece of technology and one that is easy to misuse. When the CO_2 laser is focused, it can be used for cutting skin without bleeding, and we can use this bloodless blade to treat warts, precancerous lesions, and shallow tumors. When the setting is changed to something less focused, the energy disperses to vaporize the skin's surface. A more rapidly pulsed setting is also used for a gentler facial resurfacing. Generally, I would recommend CO_2 lasers only for the most profound cases of sun damage and deep wrinkling, and treatments should be spaced 10 years apart. While some doctors argue that multiple passes with the laser create the best results, there's a greater risk of injury. Thermal damage can change the structure of the pores. A healthy pore is shaped like a goblet, but overtreatment flattens them to create an unnatural look. Overall, the skin looks smoother after the procedure, but when it's overdone, skin can look almost waxy—as if it has healed over after a burn. Some patients also experience skin discoloration.

• Erbium:YAG: This is the next generation of ablative lasers after CO_2 lasers, with a similar effect achieved in a less aggressive manner. At 2,940 nanometers, the Er:YAG wavelength penetrates the skin more gently than the CO_2 wavelength, and because it is more easily absorbed by the water that's in the skin, the heat is more scattered and the risk of thermal injury is lower. The technology also allows for more precise control in removing very thin layers of aged or damaged skin without harming surrounding healthy tissue. The cool light of the laser also causes less redness and swelling after the treatment. Er:YAG lasers are effective on mild scars, moderate facial wrinkles, and uneven skin pigment. I like them for dark, African American skin, which poses a challenge for most other laser treatments. A new generation of the technology also has a setting for a more extended pulse duration that is similar to that of the CO_2. Some laser surgeons will use a combination of both laser types, depending on the area to be treated—CO_2 for the deeper wrinkles around the eyes, mouth, and forehead and Er:YAG for the rest of the face. Skin tends to heal within 4 to 6 days with an erbium laser, versus 5 to 14 days with the CO_2. The results for Er:YAG lasers are also less dramatic, so it may not be the best choice for patients with especially deep wrinkles and folds.

THE TIGHTENERS

Recent studies show that many of the ablative laser devices just described have one very fortunate side effect: They tighten skin. But there is another, non-ablative technology that uses different types of energy—mainly radiofrequency—specifically to injure *beneath the skin* and produce a tightening effect that is the next best thing to a face-lift. Unlike the ablative lasers, these machines are designed specifically to tighten skin. Ablative lasers, which are used primarily to eradicate wrinkles and improve the overall texture of the surface of the skin, do not necessarily tighten as much as the non-ablative

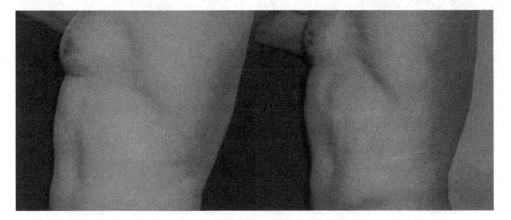

After two Thermage treatments, this patient's abs and flanks are tighter and better defined.

devices. Not all of this tightening technology is equally effective, but here is a short list of these machines and a brief description of what they can do to help give you that lift without going under the surgeon's knife:

• Thermage, which uses radiofrequency to heat cells deep below the dermis, isn't without controversy. But it remains the gold standard in nonablative treatments and is the only skin-tightening technology of its kind that's been peer-reviewed in medical journals. Thermage has seen some major new advances in recent months, and its technology is being continually improved for safety and comfort. As Samantha described in the account of her nonsurgical neck-lift, a cooling tip has dramatically reduced the burning sensation associated with treatment, enabling practitioners to use higher heat settings for greater results. A buzzing mechanism also helps

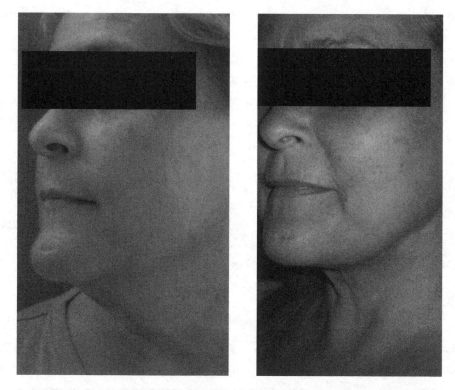

Laser lipolysis on the neck melts excess fat and tightens skin from the inside. Note the more defined and youthful appearance of this patient's jawline.

STRETCH MARKS

Do you avoid two-piece bathing suits and cover up entirely when you go to the beach or pool because of aggravated red stretch marks on your abdomen? Do you stay away from certain clothing styles because you don't want people to see the silvery stretch marks that appear on your upper arms or chest? It doesn't have to be that way anymore!

WHY DO I HAVE STRETCH MARKS?

Stretch marks are the result of a loss of the body's normal structural components, including collagen and elastin. There are five main causes of stretch marks: pregnancy, growth spurts during adolescence, heavy weight lifting, extreme weight gain/weight loss, and medications such as steroid creams or oral steroids (which can cause water retention and weight gain). Unfortunately, genetics are also responsible for determining whether you'll develop them.

HOW CAN I PREVENT STRETCH MARKS?

Prevent stretch marks during pregnancy and at other times by keeping your skin constantly well moisturized. Try to maintain a healthy, stable weight. If you're genetically susceptible to stretch marks, stay away from oral steroid medications as much as possible, and don't use potent topical steroid creams for conditions like psoriasis and eczema for prolonged periods.

WHAT CAN BE DONE ABOUT EXISTING STRETCH MARKS?

While stretch marks have been difficult to treat in the past, some good treatments are finally available that are effective in diminishing their appearance. Topical vitamin A derivatives like Retin-A or Tazorac have been shown to be effective, and some new and exciting laser-based technologies, such as the next-generation fractional lasers, can markedly improve the depressed skin, whiteness, and redness associated with stretch marks after one to three treatment sessions. Other laser technologies, including pulsed dye lasers and advanced light source technologies, have also proven helpful in making stretch marks much less visible and giving women the confidence they need to put their bikinis right back on.

distract the brain from the pain as the tip passes over particularly sensitive areas. New computer monitors have been developed that see how much heat is going under the surface of the skin and where. More targeted tips have also contributed to vast improvements in efficacy. In the hands of capable practitioners who understand how to use the technology, Thermage achieves dramatic results in patients seeking to reverse the early and middle stages of aging. New and ongoing refinements to this device are truly pushing back the need for surgery.

• EndyMed PRO by 3DEFP Technology—The latest in radiofrequency technology that just received FDA clearance. It is comprised of multiple electrodes, for more controlled delivery of heat deep into the skin, for less pain and greater protection of the overlying dermis. But it remains to be seen whether it's treatment is as powerful and effective as Thermage.

• Ulthera, which received FDA clearance in 2009, is similar to Thermage in its skin-tightening properties, but it uses focused ultrasound, which is a very new technology and an approach to skin tightening still unfamiliar to most physicians. It is also such a technique-driven technology that physicians have to treat many patients in order to get consistent results. The device has mon-

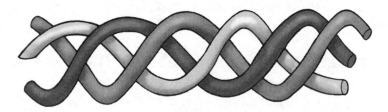

Collagen before skin-tightening treatment.

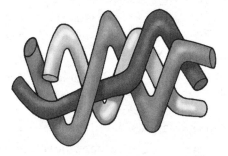

Collagen after skin-tightening treatment. Note the tighter coiling of the collagen fibers.

itors that allow doctors to see beneath the skin's surface so they can deliver non-invasive ultrasound energy at a consistent and targeted depth, thus enabling tightening of the skin. It also allows patients to be treated at two different depths, affecting twice the volume of tissue.

• Affirm also works at two levels using laser technology, claiming to tighten deep beneath the surface and improve texture at the surface level.

• Titan uses low-level infrared technology to heat and tighten the dermis, particularly for off-face areas like the abdomen, knees, arms, or elbows. It's not necessarily as powerful as other machines out there, but Titan can be good for younger patients who are just beginning to see sagging skin. However, skin-tightening results with this technology can be inconsistent, and sometimes the power is too low to produce any visible improvement.

• ReFirme combines infrared and radiofrequency energy to heat skin at medium and deep levels beneath the surface and stimulate collagen production. Billed as "a lift without a knife," it provides almost immediate effects, and improvements are significant, although not necessarily as long lasting as with Thermage.

BY A FRACTION

Fractional lasers are the next generation of ablative lasers, with the power to both resurface and tighten skin. They're called fractional because they work on microscopic treatment zones, vaporizing tissue deep within the dermis while sparing surrounding healthy tissue. This process results in immediate coagulation, tissue shrinkage, skin tightening, and surface correction. They go a step beyond IPL and CO_2 lasers because they pack just as much punch without wreaking the same kind of damage to surrounding skin cells. There are also significant tightening benefits. But, again, different machines work at different levels of efficacy.

• SmartXide is one member of the fractional laser family that uses microscopic laser dots known as DOT (dermal optical thermolysis) therapy. The

DOT laser is able to penetrate the upper layer of the dermis, which contains the most collagen, then target the water in these tissues, resulting in tissue ablation within the dot. This type of laser is particularly effective for treating scars on the face and any other area of the body. The ActiveFX and DeepFX (two different handheld devices) are both useful for treating striae, or stretch marks. ActiveFX is good for more general, surface correcting, while DeepFX can spot-treat deeper lines and scars and stimulate collagen production. Since patients usually have a combination of issues, the more options you have in one machine for customizing treatments, the better.

Patients have so many choices now when it comes to high-tech age reversal. The technologies and their results are similar—it's just a question of degree. You may want less pain and downtime and be okay with moderate results, or you may have a higher pain threshold and want maximum results. You can choose from an array of laser power, from non-ablative treatments that don't burn the skin's surface and have minimal downtime to more powerful treatments that will cause your skin to crust over as it heals. Even a single technology has multiple strengths and settings. Fraxel, which I discussed in Sarah's case study, deserves a special mention:

• Fraxel—Just as Thermage is, in my opinion, the best option for skin tightening, the Fraxel series of machines is the safest and most effective technology for laser resurfacing, with the added benefit of a little skin tightening. Microscopic laser columns, each just one-tenth the diameter of a hair follicle, penetrate deep into the dermis a fraction of tissue at a time and create tiny wounds, which trigger your body's natural response system to heal those wounds. This process expedites your body's remodeling of collagen and elastin. The technology is so precise, it's as if your skin is a digital photo that is delicately touched up one spot at a time. The laser columns stimulate a natural healing process that works from the inside out, replacing damaged tissue with younger, smoother, healthier skin. It's one of the few resurfacing lasers I recommend for darker skin because the laser isn't as strong as in the more ablative machines and it doesn't target pigment. That said, hyperpigmentation is always a risk for any patient, particularly those with olive and brown skin, because it can inflame the cells that produce melanin, although this goes away in time. Fraxel is also versatile, with three machines, each one tailor-made for different degrees of aging.

- Fraxel re:fine—The first generation and mildest version of fractional laser resurfacing for more superficial skin issues like fine lines; more of a maintenance treatment that can also help prevent the appearance of new wrinkles by stimulating collagen growth. It works best on fine lines around the eyes, age and sun spots, melasma (irregular patches of brown), and overall facial skin texture. We usually recommend four or five treatments of about 20 minutes each. There's no downtime.
- Fraxel re:store—The original machine and the technology that Sarah is using; it has minimal recovery time for a moderate effect and is great for

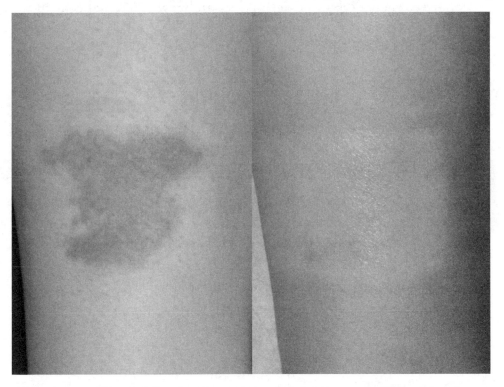

Skin abnormalities and discolorations can be completely erased with Fraxel re:store.

patients who want to soften wrinkles and correct surface imperfections like excess pigment.

- Fraxel re:pair—The second-generation, carbon dioxide–powered version; it goes much further for patients who want skin tightening as well as resurfacing. As opposed to traditional CO_2 resurfacing lasers, which vaporize and remove epidermal tissue all at once, leading to extended downtime, wound care, and a high risk of complications, Fraxel re:pair is the first CO_2 laser to treat the skin fractionally and deeply. It produces thousands of tiny wounds in the skin, penetrating much deeper than traditional ablative lasers without touching the cells around the injured area. The tissue in each of the wounds is removed with the use of the CO_2 energy. The healthy tissue surrounding the wounds then contracts, which leads to immediate tissue tightening. This spared tissue between treatment zones also promotes rapid healing while stimulating collagen production in the deep layers and new epidermal cells in the top layer. Think of it as punching hundreds of microholes into a field so that the air can get to it and the grass can grow back thicker and greener. Recovery time is about a week, much faster than with other more ablative lasers, and the procedure can actually prevent loose, sagging skin from forming.

HELLO, WORLD

Lynette, a recently divorced 40-year-old finance executive, opted for this new-generation Fraxel. She had a combination of acne scars, deep lines on her forehead and around her mouth, and some sagging around her jawline, and she wanted to give herself a dramatic makeover without surgery. She was also eager to see improvement after one treatment. Because the Fraxel laser penetrates deep into the dermis and encourages the growth of collagen, I was confident it would give her just enough of the lift she needed, along with a smoother, more perfect skin texture. But she was so eager for the treatment that I was concerned she hadn't thoroughly considered the discomfort and downtime. There would be itching, swelling, pain, and red-

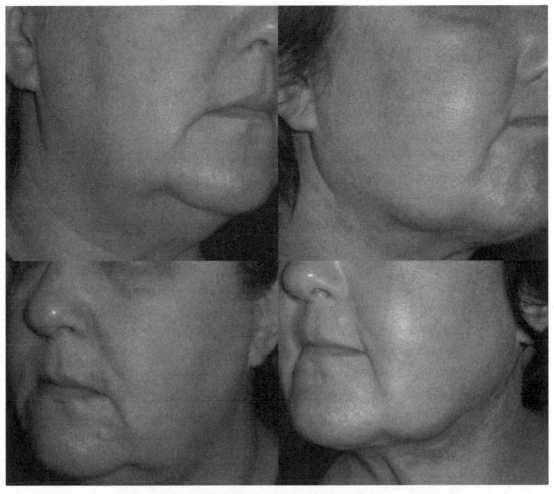

Laser liposuction can melt fat and tighten skin, even in older patients.

ness as she healed. At a minimum, she'd need to take a few days off work to recover.

"No problem, Dr. Sadick," Lynette assured me. "I did my homework and I know it won't be pleasant, but I'm prepared. Go for it!"

When she came in the following week for treatment, we gave her a Vicodin to relax her, covered her eyes with black contact lenses to protect them from the lasers, and went to work, moving the laser's tip up and down her face. She barely flinched. We sent her home with a prescription for antibiotics to prevent infection and a face full of minuscule scabs and red marks. By day four, Lynette's skin had crusted over entirely. It wasn't pretty. Healing from these procedures can be almost as uncomfortable as the downtime after traditional surgery, and patients usually try to avoid being seen in public. But by the time Lynette came to see me for a follow-up visit 2 weeks later, it was as if her beautiful, flawless face had emerged from a cocoon. The scars and lines were gone, her pores were invisible, and she had a firmness to her neck and jawline that could have rivaled that of a woman 10 years younger. The overall improvement was striking, and she was ecstatic.

"Now that I have my new face, I am finally ready for my new life. Hello, world!"

FIBER POWER

Other promising advances in lasers involve laser lipolysis for face tightening and body contouring. Yes, technically it is surgery, but of the most minimally invasive kind, with the tiniest of incisions. Laser fibers inserted via a tiny cannula under the skin apply direct heat to the deepest layers, liquefying fat, which is then extracted. New computer controls can monitor heat levels and give doctors an image beneath the surface of the skin to help them guide the laser so the procedure is much safer and the results are more consistent. For tightening a slack and puffy jawline, it is probably one of the most powerful weapons in our anti-aging arsenal. I'll discuss the benefits of laser lipolysis for off-face body shaping in Chapter 15.

The vast array of new and emerging technologies is overwhelming for patients and doctors alike, but the good news is that so much competition may eventually lower the prices of these treatments to levels more affordable for the average patient. Currently, IPL treatments cost between $300 and $600 for a single session. Ablative resurfacing treatments range between $2,000 and $3,000. Thermage, which usually takes only one treatment, ranges in price from $1,500 to $2,500. Fraxel can cost as little as $750 for the mildest treatment session to between $3,000 and $5,000 for Fraxel re:pair. Within these different types of laser treatments and machines, prices are all over the map, depending on the geography and reputation of the individual doctor.

But please, *please* be cautious about bargain hunting. As I mentioned, lasers can cause so much damage in the wrong hands, and many so-called medi-spas don't have even a dermatologist on the premises, let alone a technician who has been properly trained. Experience is key to the success or failure of these procedures. I see so many patients coming to me from other laser centers who look like burn victims, and undoing the damage involves far more work, pain, and money.

Doctors and scientists are constantly striving to develop different types of energy delivery that can safely heat the skin, circulate energy under the surface in small, targeted areas, and stimulate collagen, and newer generations of these devices are even using multiple types of energy to address various concerns in a single treatment. But at the moment, no single machine can do everything. It takes a multi-dimensional approach, and the best doctors will have more than one type of technology on their premises. The key is to keep up with the advanced generations of each machine and to learn the latest protocols for safety and efficacy. There are many ways in which all this energy interacts with tissue at multiple levels of the dermis, and the more we discover about these effects, the more we can heal and reverse the signs of aging. It's not a matter of just hitting a button or running a preset computer program; it takes commitment, time, and intense study to learn how we can best use this power to benefit our patients.

We've only just begun to scratch the surface of what this technology can do.

CHAPTER TWELVE

FINDING DR. RIGHT

IT'S NOT THE TOOLS THAT ARE THE PROBLEM—IT'S THE PEOPLE HANDLING THEM

Jacqueline is a longtime patient of mine in her early forties from Connecticut who makes her living in New York City as a real estate broker. Because she has so much day-to-day contact with the public, she's always taken care of her looks and has always been meticulous about her skin care regimen. I hadn't seen her in a while. I figured business was down with the recession, so she was skipping her usual annual treatments of filler and Botox. But it was much worse than that. When she suddenly appeared in my office recently, I barely recognized her. Jacqueline had just returned from a vacation in Saigon, Vietnam, and she looked as though she'd had way too much sun exposure. The skin on her face and neck was red and slightly blistered. I was aghast.

"What happened?" I asked her. "How could you possibly have gone to a tropical climate without wearing sunscreen and a hat? After all my warnings, didn't you know better?"

"It wasn't that, Dr. Sadick, honest," she replied. "I'm almost embarrassed to admit to you that I had a Thermage treatment while I was there. It was just so cheap!"

It turned out that Jacqueline had gone to one of the many new medi-spas cropping up in Southeast Asia to cater to a burgeoning wealthy class as well as a few foreign medical tourists looking for a deal. The place she chose was owned by a qualified doctor—at least according to the certificates he had framed in his office. His practice had been recommended by a few of Jacqueline's friends living and working as expatriates in Saigon, and the office had all the latest equipment and looked clean and well run. It seemed safe enough. But the doctor had created his own protocols—high-risk techniques that you would never see here in the United States. He believed in putting patients under with a general anesthesia so that he could blast Thermage's radiofrequency energy without the discomfort, his theory being that the more heat applied, the better the tightening effect. The problem with his rather extreme method is that patients need to be awake and able to feel some pain precisely so the doctor can know if the device is generating too much heat. With Thermage, there's a danger of overdoing the treatment and causing burning, subcutaneous fat atrophy, and long-term damage like scarring, indents, and contour depressions.

Jacqueline's surface damage was temporary and would heal soon enough, but my main concern was what was happening below the dermis. I noticed a couple of depressions in her face that were telltale signs of fat loss. Over the next few weeks, once the full extent of the injury became apparent, she would need to decide if she wanted to undergo fat grafts to even out the skin's surface and restore some of her youthful plumpness. Undoing the damage would take a lot more time, money, and pain than Jacqueline ever could have imagined.

I tried not to show it, but when Jacqueline revealed how that Saigon doctor was using Thermage, I was horrified. A few doctors in the United States had experimented with those methods more than a decade ago when the technology first came out, causing several severe injuries and warranting a lot of negative reviews. The strict protocols for using these devices in the

United States exist for a reason. While I don't doubt that there are many competent doctors practicing cosmetic dermatology outside of the United States and Europe, receiving treatments in a country where physicians have free rein with such a powerful technology is fraught with risk.

Unfortunately, Jacqueline's story is not so unusual. An increasing number of Americans are traveling abroad as medical tourists—85,000 each year, according to a recent report by McKinsey & Company—and a large chunk of the procedures they seek are cosmetic.[10] Make no mistake, some of the doctors they see are highly skilled, and the hospital facilities can be state-of-the-art. I've traveled extensively in Asia and can attest to the high level of care that's available. Bumrungrad Hospital in Bangkok, Thailand, for example, is one of the best.

But as a patient seeking treatment abroad, how can you possibly know that your physician is one of the best? There's no reliable international organization of specialists with the capacity to vet members and self-police. It's hard enough to do that state by state, let alone halfway across the world. And even if you do get the highest level of care, what about the follow-up? So much of what we do in this field involves meticulous aftercare. How well you heal from a cosmetic procedure is key to its results. If an infection, scarring, excessive bruising, or adhesions occur after you've made the return trip home, the physician who treated you is nowhere nearby. You'll have to find a local doctor and deal with the embarrassment of explaining what happened to you and where. He or she will more than likely say, "What were you thinking? Why didn't you come to me in the first place?"

It's one thing to travel abroad for a heart bypass or joint replacement because you can't afford to have it done here or your insurance does not provide adequate coverage. But a cosmetic procedure is not going to save your life, and it usually means you have some sort of discretionary income to spend on yourself, so why cut corners?

However, if you don't do your homework, you are taking just as much of a risk seeing a doctor down the street. One of the most frustrating trends in my field is that more and more patients are seeking treatment at the hands of underqualified practitioners. It hurts them and gives us qualified doctors a bad name. You do research to find the best accountant, or lawyer, or real estate agent, so why on earth wouldn't you do the same with someone who has your face and your health in his or her hands?

WORD OF MOUTH

You can find a good doctor the old-fashioned way: by word-of-mouth recommendations from friends, family, and colleagues. Ask someone you trust whom they would trust. You can also get a referral from your primary care physician. Don't set too much store by online consumer ratings of various doctors and practices. Patients have different opinions of what their doctor should be like, but medical competence is what really matters. I am continually amazed at how that comes second and third on the list when shopping for someone who is going to carry out a procedure on one of your most vital organs—your skin.

In addition to taking others' advice, you need to do your own legwork and check to see if the doctor in question is recognized by the American Board of Medical Specialties (www.certifieddoctor.org). Run that specialist's name through their database. You need to confirm that he or she isn't just a dentist who took a night course in laser peels or Botox injections. A member of the American Board of Plastic Surgery must have at least 5 years of training beyond medical school. A member of the American Academy of Dermatology must have completed a 3-year residency in dermatology and passed a rigorous two-part examination by the academy.

Bear in mind that many specialist organizations are territorial and will insist that accreditation by their specialty is the only benchmark for determining a qualified practitioner. Not necessarily. If you are having work done on your face, a maxillofacial surgeon—someone who specializes in diseases and defects of the head, neck, jaw, and mouth—may be a better bet if they've had the right training than a board-certified plastic surgeon who mostly does breast implants. In aesthetic medicine, there are about seven or eight medical specialties that are safe bets: dermatologists, cosmetic and plastic surgeons, ENT (ear, nose, and throat) specialists (because they understand the physiognomy of the face), cosmetic dentists, ophthalmologists (for the eyes), phlebologists (veins), and even a general practitioner with the right level of experience. What you want is a doctor who has an aesthetic eye, intensive training in the techniques, and a deep understanding of the physiological and anatomical structures of the face and body. The key is to match the specialty to whatever feature the doctor is treating.

And board certification isn't as important as experience, training, and patient outcomes. Even with all the right credentials, a doctor needs to have performed an adequate volume of the procedure you are seeking—at least hundreds if it involves lasers. Ideally, your practitioner will have also published an article on the treatment in a peer-reviewed journal such as the American Medical Association's *Archives of Dermatology* or have other research credentials on the subject. Reading a book on liposuction or doing a weekend workshop on laser resurfacing just won't cut it, even though the doctor is still legally allowed to perform these procedures. Research any doctors beforehand to learn where they have been accredited, what additional training and certification they've had, and how many of these procedures they perform on a regular basis. Find out if they've been involved in some of the clinical research and if the manufacturer of the device lists them as one of their recommended doctors. They have a stake in making sure the physician who recommends them has positive patient outcomes.

It also helps to know if your doctor has an affiliation at an accredited hospital, because medical colleagues will have had to approve that doctor and deem his or her qualifications acceptable. And if you are having any type of surgical procedure at an outpatient surgical center, make sure that it has been accredited by the American Association for Accreditation of Ambulatory Surgery Facilities (go to www.aaaasf.org).

Don't assume that just because something is "nonsurgical" you can safely cut corners. Deceptive advertisements and television programs promising total makeovers often give the impression that deciding to have a cosmetic procedure is as simple as buying a new shade of lipstick. There's a misconception that anyone, even a gynecologist or a dentist, can use fillers on their patients. Often they have no idea where to use it or how much to use, aesthetically or medically. So-called medi-spas also administer these treatments without an attending physician present. I see a few cases a month of botched nonsurgical treatments, including those of patients who've gone to a gynecologist for Botox and fillers, for example. The same goes for lasers. In one recent case, a woman who had faulty laser resurfacing ended up with stripes on her face. The spa technician didn't understand the protocols of the device and set the power too high, causing burns. Just because no incision or stitching is involved does not mean anyone can administer a nonsurgical cosmetic procedure.

BEWARE THE HYPE

"You want to be on the cutting edge of this field, not the bleeding edge," declared my friend and colleague Joseph Niamtu, MD, chair of the American Academy of Cosmetic Surgery Communications Committee. In other words, don't rush to try a brand-new technology. The cutting edge is something that's new but proven safe and effective. But the edge tends to get bloody when the technology just came out and nobody really knows where it is going to go. It's always exciting to witness the launch of the latest miracle machine, technique, or treatment, but if you see it on *Oprah*, it's generally wise to wait a year. We've all been guilty of getting overexcited about what's new, but consistent patient outcomes are what really matter, and that takes time to see. Remember the "thread lift"? It was all the rage in 2005, until people saw its disastrous results 1 to 2 years later. Billed as a "lunchtime lift," the thread lift ran serrated plastic sutures beneath the skin's surface in a crisscross fashion to support sagging tissue. Some patients ended up with track marks where the threads were pulling underneath the skin. Many experienced intense pain from where the barbs and threads were cutting into the dermis. And most found that the sutures didn't hold and their faces dropped after a few months. At the time, the procedure was touted on *Oprah* and many other shows as the ultimate quick fix, and it was a disaster.

Remember Moore's Law, the information technology industry maxim that technology tends to outgrow itself every 2 years? This rule applies to the machines and treatments we use in cosmetic procedures. There's always an improved version of the original laser on the horizon. Just as you shouldn't be the first to buy a new car model off the production line, neither should you be first in line to try a new medical machine until it's had a track record of success. Give us a chance to establish the best protocols and work out the bugs.

Always be especially wary when a physician or clinic is pushing one particular procedure too hard. You never know, they may simply be trying to get enough patient volume to justify the cost of the expensive piece of equipment they just bought. And don't be lured by financing deals designed to get you to sign on for a procedure you don't need and can't really afford. This is a cutthroat business, and some less scrupulous doctors in our field are using aggressive marketing tactics. But the good ones don't need to. They already get plenty of patients by word-of-mouth recommendations and because they have a rock-solid professional reputation.

Doctors love to use all the latest technology, and thousands have at least one of these new machines on their premises. But surprisingly few fully understand how each works, and the results are either minimal or damaging to patients. Let's face it, no one is immune to the ravages of lousy doctors.

As consumers seek to cut costs by going to second-rate practitioners or traveling to places like South America or Southeast Asia for bargains, there's plenty of anecdotal evidence to suggest these cosmetic horror stories are on the rise. The organizations that track procedures still show a low incidence of severe complications—at less than 1 percent, according to the American Society for Aesthetic Plastic Surgery—but that is because the society tracks only those patients of physicians accredited by their organization. The numbers do not include patients who go to their dentists for fillers, Botox, and laser treatments.[11] Not a week goes by when I don't see a woman in a state of anxiety over unforeseen side effects after having seen the wrong doctor or having her treatment administered by a nonprofessional. At best, she's wasted hundreds or thousands of dollars on something that resulted in little cosmetic improvement. At worst, she'll need to spend thousands more to fix the damage, if it can be repaired at all. And mistreatment gives the technology of lasers, ultrasound, and fillers a lousy reputation they certainly don't deserve.

It's not the tools that are the problem; it's the people handling them. If you are having a laser treatment, for example, ask questions. Find out if the doctor owns the machine or rents it. Even better, find out if he or she owns several pieces of equipment, from light-based to ultrasound and radio-wave devices. The best practitioners use several different technologies on one patient. If they have only one machine, chances are they're going to try to convince you to go with that technology even if it's not the right one for you.

You as the patient also bear some responsibility. The American Society of Plastic Surgeons recently released a survey in which 40 percent of cosmetic surgery patients claimed they should have been more proactive in learning about side effects and potential complications before surgery. Of the 301 patients polled, 80 percent were happy with the process and the results, but about a third said they experienced side effects or complications after the procedure that were "difficult to manage."[12] Among the kinds of conditions that can occur are excessive bleeding, bruising, infection, abscesses, fistulas, and slow wound healing. These incidences are generally rare, but they can happen when the patient doesn't follow his or her doctor's instructions for recovery or the doctor isn't clear enough about what should be done. And even if you don't experience side effects, your results will certainly be less than optimal. For example, cutting out cigarettes before and after a procedure is a very important advisory that certain patients simply ignore. There's only so much any physician can do when the patient doesn't take an active role in his or her own recovery.

SPILL IT!

Poor communication between doctor and patient is another hazard, and both sides are to blame. An older woman from Long Island—the aunt of one of my staff members—came to see me not long ago after turning to a number of different doctors for help. This poor lady was suffering from a severe reaction to hyaluronic acid dermal filler because she'd failed to tell her doctor that she'd had silicone injections in her face years before. Her face was subsequently broken out with several unsightly large nodules, and the fibrotic scarring was irreversible. Once I'd diagnosed her problem, all I could do was refer her to a facial plastic surgeon with experience in dealing with this type of complication. She would have to have the lumps surgically removed, a messy procedure in its own right that would lead to a different type of scarring and possibly some contour depressions. Permanent disfigurement of at least some degree was inevitable.

It's not uncommon for patients to have chronic inflammation after a silicone filler; this is one of the reasons it has fallen out of favor. It's an unpredictable material, and you can never be sure how it's going to interact with another treatment. Silicone also has a tendency to migrate, which means that it might not stay in the place it was injected. There are several cosmetic procedures that should be approached with extreme caution if you have had a silicone filler. In the case of laser treatment, for example, the silicone can act as a heat sink and cause scarring and atrophy. It's up to the doctor to quiz patients carefully about what other treatments they've had done and warn them of potential complications.

But your physician isn't a mind reader. In the case of this unfortunate patient from Long Island, the silicone filler was administered a long time ago, and she didn't remember having it. A close examination and an experienced eye should have given the doctor a clue, but it was poor communication on both sides that caused these traumatic and irreversible side effects. Don't be shy. Tell your doctor everything you think he or she needs to know, even if you find it embarrassing. This concerns your health and your beauty, so spill it!

HORROR STORIES

It's stunning to me just how reckless some practitioners are with certain treatments and how naïve their patients are about what is occurring. One of the most egregious examples was a widely reported case in 2006, when 24-year-old Fabiola DePaula died after a botched $3,000 liposuction procedure. The surgery took place in the basement of a home in Massachusetts where a Brazilian "doctor" in the United States on a 30-day work visa was performing everything from lip augmentation to nose jobs and liposuction with prescription sedatives and dirty instruments. Investigators found blood-soaked sheets and surgical equipment in a Dumpster after the doctor fled. The patient-victims were mostly immigrants from Brazil, and those who survived reported severe complications.

This is an extreme example, but skill levels in our field are all over the map, and incompetence and malpractice are more widespread than you would think. In April 2010, the FDA sent warning letters to six "medical spas" for making false or misleading claims about lipodissolve, a controversial mesotherapy treatment that injects a cocktail of chemicals subcutaneously and eliminates fat. Lipodissolve is neither widely accepted nor FDA approved, yet it is increasingly popular—especially at medi-spas, which offer the treatment along with other forms of mesotherapy. Mesotherapy is a non-surgical treatment for the removal of fat and rejuvenation of skin, employing multiple microscopic injections of pharmaceutical and homeopathic medications, plant extracts, vitamins, and other ingredients into the subcutaneous

FINDING THE RIGHT DERMATOLOGIST

A dermatologist is a physician who has completed a residency in the specialist field of dermatology, and a dermatological surgeon has completed an additional postgraduate fellowship. Qualified skin doctors should belong to either the American Society for Dermatologic Surgery or the American Academy of Dermatology. Other appropriate board memberships and certifications to look for include the following:

◆ American Board of Dermatology
◆ American Osteopathic College of Dermatology
◆ American Society for Laser Medicine and Surgery

IN CANADA:

◆ Royal College of Physicians and Surgeons of Canada
◆ Canadian Dermatology Association

fat. Unlike traditional mesotherapy, which uses more benign ingredients like nutrients and vitamins, lipodissolve uses ingredients like bile acids to cut through fatty deposits, disrupt the cell membrane, and act like a detergent to "wash" away the deposits. The body then rids itself of the cell debris and fat through urine. In theory, it's more powerful than your garden-variety mesotherapy treatment, but the lack of standardization for lipodissolve solutions and the inconsistency of injection techniques are alarming. Ingredients vary widely depending on the practitioner, and the clinical results are not all positive. It takes several weeks for fat loss to occur, and when it does, the final effect is often lumpy because the fat disappears only around the injection site. Adverse reactions also include deep, painful knots under the injection site. Patients can look and feel terrible, and there's little that can be done to smooth out the contours and reverse the indentations.

Yet medi-spa ads are everywhere touting the safety and efficacy of this procedure, comparing it with liposuction. And it's a seductive claim. Who wouldn't want to try something that melts away fat with a few injections? These are dangerous assertions, and the companies being sued by the FDA took them even further, advertising that lipodissolve can treat medical conditions like male breast enlargement, benign fatty growths, and surgical deformities.

Mesotherapy is an option worth considering for nonsurgical body contouring and localized fat loss for reasons I will discuss in Chapter 15. Trials are under way to improve the standardization of formulas and treatment techniques, but for now, patients should be wary of overhyped claims and seek out only the most experienced practitioners with proven results, as this is a heavily technique-dependent procedure. The only real protection you have as a consumer is to be well-informed.

YOUR RIGHT TO KNOW

When you choose a doctor, demand to see before and after pictures of his or her patients. Lots of them. And take the time to conduct an interview. Here is a list of questions you should ask your dermatologist or plastic surgeon (and if he or she is reluctant or hesitant to answer, go elsewhere):

- How many procedures like mine have you performed?

- Do you own or rent your equipment?

- Will you be performing the procedure yourself, or will it be one of your nurses or a medical assistant?

- What are the risks associated with this type of procedure?

- What are the alternative treatments?

- Is there anything that you suggest I do before the procedure to ensure better results and a quicker recovery?

- What will the recovery be like?

- How soon before I can see results?

- When can I begin wearing makeup and using skin care products again?

- For how long should I avoid the sun?

- When can I begin exercising?

- How can I maintain the results?

There are no shortcuts. If the treatment is cheap, there's a reason for it, and you'll end up paying more to undo the damage. After getting burned—literally and figuratively—it may take you a long time to consider other procedures to effectively turn back the clock. You lose out twice: first from the mess made by an underqualified practitioner and a second time when you shy away from all the amazing advances that can restore your youth in the hands of Dr. Right.

CHAPTER THIRTEEN

PLUMP UP THE VOLUME

NATURAL BEAUTY AT THE END OF A NEEDLE

Victoria was a self-described "cosmetic procedure virgin." She was an extremely fit yoga fanatic in her mid-fifties who took great care of her skin and stayed out of the sun, but beyond investing in a few decent department store moisturizers, she hadn't even had so much as a facial. She didn't start wearing makeup until she turned 50, and the idea of injecting a foreign substance into her face appalled her. She'd joke with her husband and friends about those poor ladies who'd so obviously had too much cosmetic and surgical enhancement. She vowed never to be one of those victims of vanity.

But when she looked in the mirror, she could see more lines forming on her forehead and around her eyes. She started to feel that her face was looking gaunt. With growing curiosity, she regarded magazine articles about the latest fillers and nonsurgical treatments. Then a friend in her book club showed up for a meeting looking inexplicably fresh and well rested. Victoria asked what she was up to, thinking she must have just returned from a spa vacation. She was shocked to learn that this friend had just had her face strategically "plumped" with Restylane, one of the most popular hyaluronic acid (HA) dermal fillers. (HA is produced naturally by the body and acts as a humectant, binding with water and plumping up the skin, almost like a sponge.) That did it. Victoria did some research and made an appointment with me the following week, "just to see."

I could tell right away that a little more volume would do wonders for Victoria's appearance. She had smooth skin, great bone structure, and very few lines for a woman her age, but because she had so little body fat, her midcheek area was hollow, and the area under her eyes, her tear troughs, needed more volume. Her nasolabial folds also needed some softening.

We started with a little Botox around the brows, in the corners of her eyes, and at her jawline to help pull up sagging skin. We waited a few days for it to kick in. The advantage of treating the face with neurotoxin before using filler is that it helps immobilize certain facial muscles, which in turn enables the filler agent to stay in place and form a kind of scaffolding to support the upper layers of the skin. When Victoria returned with a dramatically smoother brow, we went to work on certain key areas of her face that needed added thickness.

I used Perlane, another gel-based HA filler. It's made by the same company that developed Restylane and contains the same ingredients, but it is formulated thicker so it can be placed deeper in the dermis and potentially last a bit longer. I knew Victoria was nervous. I wanted to make sure that we took a very conservative approach that would last only 6 to 8 months and would be easily reversible with an antidote if for any reason Victoria was unhappy with the results. That way, she could get used to the idea of having filler in her face and opt for something more long lasting once the effects of the Perlane wore off.

The other advantage of Perlane is that it doesn't require any pre-testing on the patient's skin. It's a natural body chemical that fills up the skin like

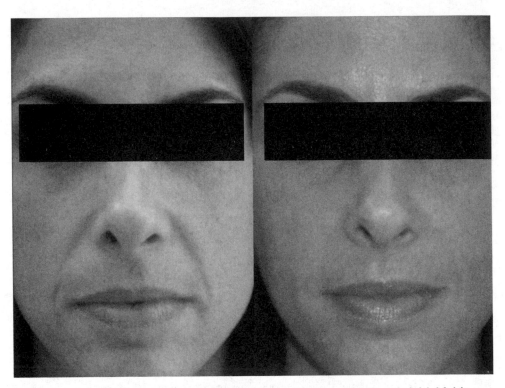

A single Perlane treatment dramatically softened this patient's nasolabial folds.

normal tissue, and its soft, gel-like texture also makes it easy to mold and contour to the face for a subtle effect. It was enough to noticeably soften Victoria's laugh lines, and the added volume near her tear troughs helped to decrease the darkness under her eyes and give her a brighter, more rested look. I also added some of the filler above the border of her upper lip to give more definition to the lip line and smooth out some feathery lines that were starting to appear.

We sent Victoria home with some ice packs and a tube of arnica gel to help with the slight bruising that sometimes occurs at the injection sites. She didn't want to tell her husband what she had done, so she timed her visit to us while he was away on a business trip and worked from home for the next couple of days. A week later, she came for her follow-up visit and she looked fantastic. Her skin looked rested and glowing in the most natural way possible. Victoria confessed that she couldn't stop looking at herself in the mirror, she was so pleased. Her husband was none the wiser, but he kept commenting on how good she looked. She caught a couple of the ladies in her book club giving her some admiring and curious stares, but they never asked, and she never told them.

A year later, Victoria came back to see me, but this time she asked for a longer-lasting filler, along with a few more of the anti-aging treatments we talk about in this book, such as Thermage, to tighten her skin, and a laser peel to deal with some age spots. Fillers were her first step into the wonderful world of age reversal at its most natural and subtle. She realized that she didn't have to end up looking like a chipmunk with a mouthful of nuts. She could have the best of both worlds, with more fullness in her face and a natural range of facial expression.

"I finally understand that this is part of the maintenance plan, like eating right and doing yoga," she enthused. "This is just another way I can continue to look like my best self. And no one else needs to know!"

Millions of women, and men, are making the same discovery about fillers. It's one of the safest and easiest ways to combat the signs of aging. Hyaluronic acid dermal fillers were rated number two of the top five nonsurgical procedures in 2007, for a total of almost 1.5 million procedures, according to the American Society for Aesthetic Plastic Surgery.[13] These numbers will increase dramatically as more kinds of dermal fillers become approved by the FDA and more patients seek out nonsurgical solutions to combat wrinkles, folds, and loss of volume.

New-generation fillers are among the most powerful tools in our anti-aging arsenal. They can give you a key marker of youth that not even the most skilled plastic surgeon can offer: volume. They can erase those deep folds around the mouth and smooth out tired, hollow eyes. They can give a sunken face all the fullness of baby fat. They can give structure and thickness to the skin, sculpting and correcting the planes of the face to subtly reverse time by 5 to 10 years.

But when they are administered clumsily, fillers can have an unfortunate and unflattering effect. We've all seen those actresses who went too far, had too much injected in the lower half of the face, and wound up with bizarrely distorted features. As with anything, ease of use tempts some doctors, and patients, to take it too far. But when these agents and fillers are used correctly, they can build volume to the entire structure of the face for an incredibly natural and long-lasting effect. As discussed, they can even be used on off-face areas, like the chest and hands, or to even out surface depressions caused by cellulite or post-liposuction defects.

Not all fillers are created equal. Some are too thick for the more delicate areas of the face. Others don't last long enough. What I look for in filler is safety, ease of use, longevity, and consistency of results. The ideal injectable filler remains elusive to this day, although I do have my biases. We've come a long way from the days of liquid silicone and implants. But I won't be satisfied until we can develop filler that can last for years and keep the skin tissue of the face constantly producing new collagen. With the advent of stem cell technology, it's just on the horizon.

There is a wide and ever-expanding array of choices, and the trick is finding the right filler for your individual needs and expectations. Some prefer a subtle, more gradual effect, while others want an "instant face-lift." A longer-lasting product may be a priority for those who don't want to keep coming back every 8 to 12 months for injections, while others may not mind regular maintenance as long as the substance used is safe and biocompatible. Cost may be another factor. The price per syringe can vary between $500 and $1,000, and sometimes a patient may need as many as three syringes, depending on the size and shape of the face and the areas to be treated. Be wary if the price of materials on offer is too much of a bargain, because some less scrupulous physicians dilute the formula. You might as well be throwing your money away, because the effect won't last, and the physician may be using more vials of the weakened filler, so you will be paying more anyway. It's such a widespread practice that the American Society of Plastic Surgeons recently issued a public warning to consumers looking to cut costs during the economic downturn. Patients run real safety risks for the sake of bargain basement pricing, including getting filler treatments at their gynecologist's or dentist's office. It is truly a case of getting what you pay for. Using filler is already a more economical option than getting a face-lift, so don't be cheap. This is your face, your calling card to the rest of the world.

Doctors may also push for a particular brand of filler simply because they have a relationship with the manufacturer. We all work with developers and manufacturers of new treatments and technology, and some of us have our particular favorites, often with good reason. But make sure your doctor discloses that relationship and lays out several options during the consultation. It goes without saying that whoever administers the filler should be a qualified plastic surgeon or cosmetic dermatologist with experience performing a high volume of these procedures. And whatever their credentials and experience, don't take their word for it when it comes to the right filler for you. It always helps to arm yourself with the correct and most up-to-date information before you make that appointment, so read on!

IN THE BEGINNING

The now notorious liquid silicone was first injected as a filler around 1950. It is permanent, doesn't produce the most naturalistic effect, and can cause potential complications, including infections and the fact that the outer layers of skin can drape differently over the silicone substance as the face ages. The result can be less than aesthetically pleasing. Silicone has also been known to migrate to different areas, potentially creating an abnormal appearance. And if you're not happy, the only way to get rid of it is to have it surgically removed, which totally defeats the purpose of nonsurgical filler.

Bovine-based collagen came about in 1981, but some patients were allergic, and the volumizing effects lasted for only a few months. More recent variations of collagen filler are CosmoDerm and CosmoPlast, human collagen with fewer side effects. But today, even in these newer brands, collagen is thought of as a thing of the past. It works pretty well as a filler and may last a little longer than hyaluronic acid–based fillers, but you won't find many doctors who offer it. Overall, there are better products out there now. We've moved on.

Another original breed of filler I have mentioned is your own fat, transferred from another part of your body, like your thighs or love handles, through a minor liposuction procedure. I really like the naturalistic effect of this procedure. Your own fat has the perfect consistency for use elsewhere on your body, and it's the safest of all the fillers because it's not synthetic. And you can't find a substance that is more biocompatible than your own tissue. But consistency of results is a problem. Fat globules are harder to control and tend to migrate, and there is always a risk of injury or infection when a skin incision is involved. Once the fat is extracted, you may want to have your doctor store any leftovers, because in less than 6 months the fat will be reabsorbed by your body and the plumping effect will be long gone. For this reason, unless you introduce fat stem cells, fat transfers may not be worth the effort and expense.

Hyaluronic acid fillers are the most widely offered these days, and their use exploded when the first version, Restylane, was approved by the FDA in 2003. Derived from animal sources, each of these products has subtle differences and varying concentrations of HA, but they tend to have fewer side effects than other fillers, are easier to use, and are quickly reversible with the injection of an antidote called hyaluronidase. This is a key advantage, because it allows physicians to reverse and adjust the look if the patient isn't happy and feels the filler was overdone in certain places. It's also a great safeguard in the event of an adverse reaction. Studies at University of Michigan Medical School found that hyaluronic acid fillers can lead to collagen production and slow the breakdown in your own collagen reserves.[14] More research is needed, and it's not exactly clear how much collagen is produced or how long it lasts, but this could be an added bonus for regular users of HA fillers over time.

There are now dozens of HA-based fillers on the market. Costs per syringe vary depending on the location and the doctor. Here are a few that you are most likely to see advertised in your dermatologist's waiting room:

• Restylane (by Medicis Aesthetics)—Again, this was the first to be FDA approved. It works best for filling middle to deep areas below the dermis and smoothing out wrinkles, nasolabial folds, crow's-feet, and forehead lines. It's also commonly used to plump up facial hollows and to fill those depressions around the eyes known as orbital troughs, although I find in some patients this causes a bluish discoloration under the eyes, particularly if the injection is too close to the surface. The substance is a little too thick to go deep and close enough to the orbital bone to fill out the tear troughs, although some physicians do like using it around the eye. It generally takes 2 to 3 days for mild bruising and swelling to settle down, and the plumping effects usually wear off after 6 months. Side effects are minimal, and allergic reactions and complications are relatively rare. However, about 1 in 2,000 patients suffer extreme tenderness, redness, and bumps. If you have herpes simplex, be warned that Restylane can trigger an outbreak, especially around the mouth. (Costs between $300 and $800 per vial.)

• Perlane—Also made by Medicis Aesthetics, Perlane was approved by the FDA in 2007 and is similar to its predecessor, Restylane, except that it's designed to reach deeper into the dermis and fill out deeper skin folds and depressions. In Perlane, more molecules of hyaluronic acid are clumped together, which makes it denser than Restylane. It also takes a little longer to metabolize and therefore lasts longer. Its gel particles are particularly good for filling out the midcheek area, and it can also be used for augmenting the chin and firming the jawline to lift sagging jowls. Side effects are equally minimal. Depending on the areas of the face that need correcting, your doctor may opt to use both products—Restylane for superficial fine lines and Perlane for deep filling. Be aware that if an unskilled practitioner injects Perlane too close to the surface, it could create a lumpy effect. Make sure your physician has been using this substance on a high volume of patients. (Costs between $500 and $900 per vial.)

• Juvéderm (by Allergan)—FDA approved in 2006, this variation on HA fillers consists of more homogeneous particles than competing brands like Restylane, which means it can take longer to break down and therefore last longer, although this remains unproven. HA concentrations vary according to the different formulations, including Juvéderm Ultra and Juvéderm Ultra Plus, which are designed to be used as volumizing agents at varying depths below the dermis and are now under FDA investigation. (Costs between $400 and $900 per vial.)

• Prevelle Silk—FDA approved in 2008, this is the least expensive of the HA family of fillers, with one of the lowest concentrations of the acid. It lasts only a couple of months. Some doctors like it because it gives nervous patients a chance to try out a temporary filler. It also contains the numbing agent lidocaine, and thanks to its lower concentrations of ingredients, it requires only a small-gauge needle to be administered. (Costs between $200 and $600 per vial.)

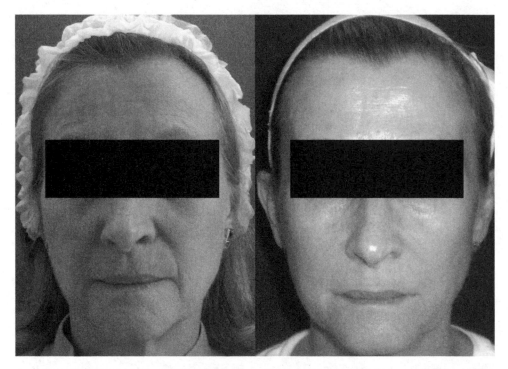

A combination of HA fillers with Radiesse were injected into this patient's lower cheeks to globally rejuvenate her entire face.

Newly approved versions of Juvéderm, Restylane, and Perlane also contain lidocaine, although some doctors prefer to mix a numbing agent in addition to a topical numbing cream and nerve blockers. It depends on the pain tolerance of the patient and the sensitivity of the area to be filled. Dozens more HA-based fillers are on the verge of FDA approval. There's little to distinguish these brands, but competition on the market is a good thing for patients because it will lower the cost of these fillers dramatically.

Besides the hyaluronic acid–based fillers, other, longer-lasting fillers have recently been approved by the FDA. Artefill is the only FDA-approved filler that is permanent. Artefill was launched on the market in 2006 and claims to last as long as 10 years without the need for touch-ups, and doctors in Europe who have been using the filler for a few years longer are finding this is truly the case. Though Artefill is still living down a bad reputation from problems early on in its use, the newer formulations are much improved. About 20 percent of Artefill consists of PMMA, or poly(methyl methacrylate), a material used to make Plexiglas but also used safely in medicine for the last half century. The PMMA in Artefill consists of highly polished—but very tiny—microspheres suspended in purified bovine collagen. A small amount of lidocaine is also in the mix. A nice bonus to the filling effect is that it stimulates collagen growth, which is an additional reason it is so long lasting. But Artefill's longevity and viscosity are also its drawbacks. While it's great for filling out deep wrinkles, folds, and scars, it's not a product for filling out near thin skin under the eyes, at the temples, or around the neck. And patients with generally thin, delicate skin should not choose Artefill.

It's worth pointing out once more that the more permanent the filler, the more it behooves you to find the best practitioner possible. Take a look at as many before and after photos of actual patients as you can, be very specific about the areas you want to fill, and express exactly how subtle, or dramatic, you want the effect to be.

For deep furrows and wrinkles, Radiesse may be better than most of the other filler options. It comprises minute particles, or microspheres, of calcium hydroxylapatite (the mineral found in tooth enamel). This material is suspended in a gel-like compound, giving it a unique thickness and elasticity. Because of its texture, Radiesse can be injected into a deeper plane of the face, then molded for several minutes after injection to smooth out the contour. Clinical tests have shown that Radiesse, like Artefill, can stimulate new collagen growth in injected areas. It also lasts 8 to 12 months. But Radiesse is not ideal for use around the eyes, where the skin is too thin and delicate and the injector won't be able to go deep enough for a subtle effect. It works best on more severe signs of aging, to fill out those marionette lines that are stubbornly resistant to other fillers, and is an excellent agent for augmenting localized facial volume. It's also cost-effective for patients because it lasts for more than a year and there's more material in each syringe than there would be for less viscous fillers like those that are hyaluronic acid based, so you don't need to use as much.

For the most naturalistic volumizing effect, I usually recommend Sculptra, a compound I have already mentioned several times in this book. This filler was approved by the FDA for cosmetic purposes in summer 2009 and is only just beginning to see widespread use. But next to fat, it's become one of my top choices for building volume and smoothing out lines in most areas of the face, even under the eyes. The active ingredient is poly-L-lactic acid, a synthetic polymer derived from the alpha hydroxy acid family and used in solid form as fibers for sutures in many common surgical procedures. It was first used on HIV patients to correct facial wasting. Sculptra's side effects are minimal, the solution is easy to mold, and it has been proven to thicken skin over time by stimulating collagen.

The whole point of Sculptra is that it works gradually, for noticeable results that emerge subtly over the course of two to three treatments and can last up to 2 years or more. When Sculptra is mixed with the new cell therapy solutions, such as platelet-rich plasma, effects can last even longer. But, as with all of the best anti-aging solutions, it requires a little patience. It takes many years for your face to age, so if you want to reverse that damage and still look human, don't expect it to happen overnight. If you'd like to be discreet with others about any cosmetic procedures you've had done, a slower, more subtle improvement takes a lot less explaining than some-

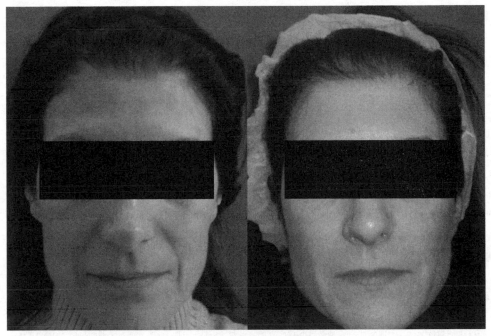

Sculptra is an ideal filler for revolumizing the mid-face and correcting dark circles and hollowness around the eyes. This patient had a series of Sculptra treatments four to six weeks apart.

thing more dramatic. People will notice you look great, but they won't necessarily know why.

Because it's so natural looking, I particularly like Sculptra for men. Nathan, a patient I had, just wanted an overall global improvement to his skin, to "freshen" him up. I recommended Sculptra because I knew Nathan would appreciate its gradual, natural rejuvenating effect. While it can target specific areas, it's also great as a general volumizer. I've used it on myself, and I've been thrilled with the results.

TOUGH CUSTOMER

Nathan was one of my more challenging customers. A ruggedly handsome New Yorker, he wasn't the type you'd imagine would seek out cosmetic treatments,

FILLER FINE POINTS

◆ Seek out a board-qualified dermatological, plastic, or cosmetic surgeon who understands the musculature of the face to perform the procedure.

◆ Make sure the doctor has expertise in using more than one kind of filler.

◆ Bring a picture of yourself looking your best to give your doctor an idea of the end result you are going for.

◆ Ask to see before and after pictures of other patients.

◆ If it's your first time seeking a filler, or you are trying a new doctor, go for a filler that doesn't last as long, and be conservative in how much you use.

◆ Use Botox alongside filler to bolster and prolong the effect.

although there was a reason he looked so good for his 56 years. Nathan was a professional musician and soap actor; his livelihood depended on looking good, and he'd taken meticulous care of his appearance. With another doctor, he'd had his own fat injected into his eye and upper cheek areas every 2 years. Occasionally, he'd alternate these treatments with Restylane, but he was never entirely satisfied with the results. A decade before he came to see me, he'd even had an operation on his lower lids. As a result, he'd lost volume and was starting to get a hollowed-out look under his eyes. I told him we could fix that by injecting Sculptra deep under the muscle, close to the orbital bone.

"I'm not sure I believe you, Doc," he declared. "I was told you can't get that close."

Not every doctor has the deftness of touch to get close enough to the delicate eye area, but I assured him I could certainly get close enough to give him some volume under his eyes and fix the problem.

On the day of the procedure, Nathan was nervous. We covered the injection sites (the lower two-thirds of his face) with numbing cream. He fired questions at us about how it would work. Sculptra wasn't the same type of filler he was used to. Unlike hyaluronic acid fillers, Sculptra isn't a one-shot deal. The collagen grows gradually, and you focus on certain areas over the course of three treatments, set 4 to 6 weeks apart. These intervals allow you to build up a base of your own collagen, to which you add layers, sculpting the face underneath the musculature as you go. It's like sowing seeds and waiting for them to sprout, then continuing to cultivate. When the procedure is done right, I've seen the effects last for a few years.

I gave Nathan about 12 shots on each side of his face, focusing on his lower mandible, to build up his jawline and correct some slight sagging, and his midcheek area to fill out the planes of his face. It's essential to take a different approach when working with men. You can soften the effect of the nasolabial folds, but never too much, because character lines are more masculine. If you go too far and smooth them out completely, you'll end up with a monkey face. Overall, the injections should follow a squarish pattern on men, as opposed to a heart-shaped outline for women. Too often, doctors use an identical approach on both sexes, and the men end up with oddly feminized features. This can happen when physicians don't really look at their patients or ask about their expectations.

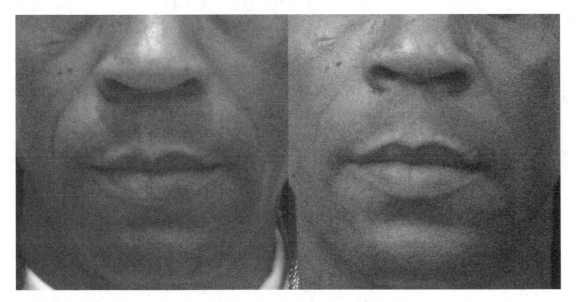

Even in men, volumizing fillers can create subtle but noticeable improvements around the mouth, jawline, and mid-face.

Nathan was extremely impatient to see the results. After about a week, the bruising under his eyes dissipated, and so did the swelling. He concluded the procedure hadn't worked for him. Six weeks later, after some prodding from his wife (that's usually what it takes), Nathan came in to see me for a follow-up treatment. I could already see a substantial improvement, but he told me he felt he was wasting his time and money. Of course, he quickly changed his tune when he saw his own before and after photos and willingly returned again for a third treatment. It wasn't just the structure of his face that improved, but the overall tone and texture of his skin. We are not certain why yet, but Sculptra somehow imparts a healthy, youthful glow to the skin's surface.

A year later, Nathan still looks great, not a day over 45. I made a believer out of a hard-nosed skeptic.

"You were right, Doc," he said. "Coming in three times for treatments was a hassle, and the bruising was no picnic, but in the end it was well worth it."

FILLER FRONTIER

Used wisely, volumizing and filling products work deep under the dermis to build a kind of "scaffolding" to fight sagging and stimulate fibroblasts. But it takes a multifaceted approach, combining microscopic injections for fine lines and scars and deeper injections to build overall volume into the face.

This area of cosmetic dermatology is constantly improving. We're seeing increasing trends toward fillers with larger molecules that can create friction under the skin for biostimulation of fibroblast and collagen growth. Early studies suggest these filling agents can induce almost as much remodeling of the dermis as the heat produced by laser and radiofrequency technology. Dermal thickening may also be possible, although we need more ongoing, long-term studies to prove these claims.

The more we study the process of photoaging, the more we have come to understand that it is not just about age spots, lines, and wrinkles, but also about volume loss within the entire structural anatomy of the face. That's why the best approach to take with fillers is a holistic one, penetrating to the deeper structures of the face through layers of fat and muscle tissue and even to the bone.

Future generations of fillers may turn out to be hybrid products that work synergistically to address both the more superficial wrinkles and deeper issues such as a general loss of volume and depressions in the face. Combinations of collagen or hyaluronic acid with calcium molecules are already being explored. This is a constantly evolving field where the treatment options just get better and better. We may yet find the perfect permanent filler that's both biocompatible and completely reversible. One of the most simple, effective, and dramatic solutions for aging is waiting for us at the tip of a needle. Stay tuned!

CHAPTER FOURTEEN

HAIR-APY

YES, WE WILL CURE BALDNESS ONE DAY

No top-to-toe beauty book would be complete without addressing hair loss, one of the most devastating signs of aging that can strike at any time.

When my patient Maggie started losing clumps of her hair at the age of 30, she got creative to keep it a secret. A real estate broker who dealt with the public all the time, she constantly worried, "Did they see my spot? Is it still covered?" She wore wigs and hairpieces, doing anything she could to camouflage her baldness. Maggie also tried several treatments. Some of them helped, but not enough. She saw specialist after specialist. Finally, we determined the cause of her hair loss to be inflammation due to an underlying autoimmune disorder. Somehow, Maggie had developed antibodies in her hair follicles, and her immune system was engaging in friendly fire against her own hair, preventing growth. By the time she got to me, she was an emotional wreck.

"Dr. Sadick, this is the worst thing that's ever happened to me. I feel like less of a woman. I have nightmares about my wig falling off and people seeing what's underneath. I live in perpetual fear of humiliation."

I sympathized. While growing bald is traumatic enough for men, for women it can be utterly devastating. Thirty million, or one in five, women in the United States suffer from hair loss—almost equivalent to the number of men—and this loss is usually caused by aging, illness, genetics, or hormonal changes after menopause. Sometimes the hair loss is due to a combination of these factors. But the earlier it can be treated, the better the chances of halting its progress and even restoring some hair growth.

We started Maggie on a topical treatment using a steroid-infused lotion in combination with minoxidil, a custom prescription formulation I use in my practice. This solution works on hair follicles to reverse the shrinking process of the follicle and stimulate new growth on the top of the scalp. Within 4 months, Maggie's hair grew back thick and lush, and she hasn't worn a wig since.

"Having my hair back has changed my whole outlook on life," Maggie told me on a follow-up visit. "I feel feminine again. You gave back a part of me I thought I'd lost forever."

Maggie was fortunate. Not everyone can regrow their lost hair, and even if they manage to find their way to one of the few true experts in hair loss scattered across the country, it may be too late to help them. This is an exciting new frontier exploding with possibility, but right now the best we can do for most men and women is to stop the hair loss in its tracks with light therapies, topical treatments, and, if it's gone that far, hair transplants. If hair thinning and shedding haven't progressed too far, it can be stopped in its tracks and patients are able to keep what hair they do have—infinitely better than losing it all.

I should know. My hair started to fall out when I was just a teenager. Every man in my family experienced early hair loss, but I couldn't accept it. It felt as if I were losing my identity, and I was determined to do something about it. At 18, I did my research and discovered a pioneering surgical program for hair transplants. I was one of the first people in the country to receive this treatment, and those early 1970s methods were crude. I was butchered. Pieces of my scalp were taken from the back of my head, and I experienced profuse bleeding and intense pain. But it was no comparison to the emotional devastation I felt when I saw the final result—a scalp full of neat rows of tufts that looked exactly like doll's hair. There was nothing natural about it.

I've had to live with that disaster ever since. There's nothing I can do about it. I keep my hair short and pray that the first thing people notice about me is my face and my healthy, youthful skin. But who am I kidding? Hair is everything. Throughout the centuries, people have been obsessed with hair. A healthy head of lush, shiny strands is a marker of youth and a symbol of sensuality. For a man, it represents virility. For a woman, it's a huge part of her beauty and sexual identity.

Not so when you are bald or balding. Not only is it an obvious marker of aging, in many cultures it is even a stigma to have no hair. In the past, societies have shaved the heads of prisoners and traitors as a mark of shame. The Romans used to cut the hair of women found guilty of adultery. Monks and nuns of all religions, from Buddhism to Catholicism, shave their heads to make them less sexually attractive. What does that tell you?

I've lost count of how many women have sat in my office sobbing because they have thinning hair and bald patches. Hair loss is a taboo subject among women, and many people assume it's not an issue. It takes a long time for patients to get the information they need, if they ever find it. And only those lucky enough to have the resources get the kind of treatment they need.

You'd be surprised by how few physicians pay attention to hair, even though hair follicles can say a lot about a person's internal health. Women and men come to me from all over the country and all over the world to seek treatments for hair loss. They've heard about my research. I have served on the board of examiners for the International Society of Hair Restoration Surgery and as a member of the Scientific Advisory Council of the Hair Research Foundation, so it's my business to know what's cutting-edge in hair loss. By the time patients see me, they have often already experienced a series of confusing or inaccurate diagnoses and ineffective treatments from other doctors. I am their last best hope. But the good news is that there *is* hope.

ROOT CAUSES

The key to treating hair loss in both men and women is to understand its root causes. Contrary to popular assumptions, hair loss is not solely a matter of genetics. Nor is hair loss inevitable as we age. Some forms of hair loss are temporary conditions that may eventually cure themselves, while others are more complex—associated with disease, inflammation, autoimmune conditions, and other systemic disorders such as viral infections and fungal diseases. Knowing the cause is the first step to finding the cure. Like skin, hair is a great diagnostic tool. When you take care of your crowning glory and are alert to changes and signs, you are also taking care of your overall health. Here's what to look for:

• **Androgenetic Alopecia**—Known as male pattern baldness, this is the most common cause of hair loss and the one that receives the most attention. It affects 30 million men in the United States, and 95 percent of this hair loss is linked to genetics. The hair loss itself usually starts in the second decade of life and continues with increasing persistence. The second warning sign is a noticeable thinning of scalp hair. The receding hairline eventually forms a horseshoe pattern, with a remaining fringe along the sides of the scalp. The hair follicles are not gone forever, but they've become fine, blond, babylike hairs, like the kind you'd see on an infant's scalp.

• **Women's Androgenetic Alopecia**—Known as female pattern or genetic balding, this type of hair loss is triggered by hormones. The degree of loss is usually not as extensive as it is in the male population, though, because of the

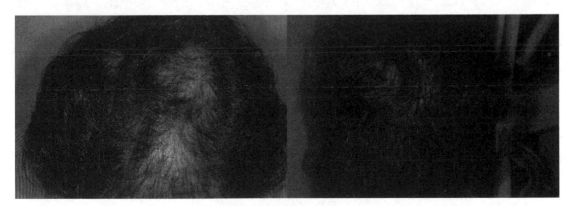

After two LED red light laser treatments and a follicular unit transplant, this early stage case of male pattern baldness is all but reversed.

protection provided by estrogen. The hair loss develops much more slowly and later in life and tends to result in a diffuse thinning all over the scalp rather than actual baldness. Most women can tell by the texture and body that it's not the hair it used to be, and it eventually reaches the point where they begin to see scalp and not hair. Women tend to get a round or oval-shaped area right behind the hairline that gets very thin, and it's often at that point that they seek treatment. But women who begin to shed their hair in this pattern, particularly quickly, should consult their physicians right away, because the cause may be something other than genetics. It could be triggered by adrenal and ovarian diseases, an iron deficiency, hypothyroidism, hyperthyroidism, or various kinds of tumors that increase hormone levels, including testosterone. Antidepressants, both types of blood pressure medication—beta-blockers and calcium channel blockers—and antianxiety medications can also exacerbate hair loss in women with a genetic predisposition. Even a nonsteroidal anti-inflammatory like Motrin or Advil can worsen the condition. A smart internist or dermatologist will run a series of blood tests to rule out the sometimes serious health issues that can cause hair loss.

• **Temporary Hair Loss**—There is a natural life cycle to the hair follicle. Human hair grows only to a certain length over several years and is then shed. A biological clock is built into every strand of hair, so that it doesn't all shed and renew itself at the same time. But certain external factors can override this cycle and affect large numbers of hair follicles at the same time. The hair goes into a resting or shock phase after any type of physiological insult. The condition is called telogen effluvium, and it is almost always temporary. When a woman becomes pregnant, for example, her hair often remains longer than normal in an active growing state as a result of pregnancy hormones, but after childbirth, that hair enters a reduced or resting phase for 3 to 6 months and the new mother may experience extensive hair loss. Babies also shed scalp hair in their first 6 months and appear entirely bald until they grow in permanent hair. Adults, however, can lose as much as 50 percent of their hair in an affected area before even noticing the hair loss. Certain traumas and drugs can also trigger telogen effluvium in both men and women, including fever, surgery, severe infection, chronic illness, and endocrine disorders. Ingested vitamin A derivatives, blood thinners like heparin, anticonvulsants, certain antithyroid drugs, and even increased levels of heavy metals like lead and arsenic in the blood can cause hair loss. Women who are on crash diets and lose a great deal of weight over a short period of time have also been known to shed profuse amounts of hair. Anything that puts physical stress on the body and causes it to recycle its hair into a resting phase can lead to temporary hair loss. But once the physical condition that causes the hair loss is removed, the hair can regrow in 6 to 12 months.

• **Alopecia Areata**—Immunologic hair loss occurs when inflammatory diseases cause a person's immune system to become overactive. This condition decreases the number of peripheral blood cells that help regulate and control immunologic activity. It's not at all unusual. At least 0.5 percent of new patients in dermatologists' offices have the disease, and by the age of 50 at least 1 percent of the population will have experienced immunologic hair loss at some point in their lives. Areata is Latin for "round" or "circumscribed," which means that people suddenly see oval-shaped bald spots here or there or tiny short hairs that are broken off. Sometimes it's noticed by the person cutting their hair. There may be underlying genetic causes for this condition. We've seen cases of identical twins developing alopecia simultaneously, and the condition can run through three or four generations in families. Hair falls out, leaving behind soft white skin totally devoid of hair. Other patterns in alopecia include a band of rimmed hair loss along the scalp margin, the loss of scalp hair, or the loss of body and scalp hair. Hair changes its pigment, and fingernails and toenails can show stippling or grooves. The condition is benign, but it's hard to predict, and its rapid onset can be extremely distressing to patients. It can be a chronic condition, with hair growth on some parts of the body and continued hair loss in other areas, or it can be short-lived and acute. It can stabilize for years or progress within a matter of weeks. In about half of alopecia areata cases the attacks last for less than a year, and in about 70 percent of cases the condition is resolved within 5 years. But for the remaining 30 percent of alopecia areata sufferers, the prognosis is poor. And science hasn't determined the exact cause. It may be partly hereditary, and the most recent evidence suggests the main trigger is an autoimmune disorder that causes the body's immune system to attack hair follicles and disrupt hair's normal formation. Allergies, thyroid disease, ulcers, vitiligo, lupus, and rheumatoid arthritis can all be triggers. But the good news with this condition is that for most, there is always the possibility for regrowth, even in cases of total baldness.

Other rare conditions and circumstances can cause or worsen hair loss, but most are eminently treatable. A less common cause is bacterial infection. *Staphylococcus aureus,* the most common cause of staph infections, can produce abscesses deep in the hair follicle. The infection is usually spread by contaminated hands and mostly affects those whose immune systems are compromised, like the sick and the elderly, although 20 percent of the population are carriers. The good news is that the bacteria can be treated with the appropriate antibiotics. Carbuncles, or infections of multiple connecting hair follicles, occur in the elderly and can be associated with diabetes and cardiac failure or the use of immune-suppressing drugs. But they are treatable with steroids. Syphilis and tuberculosis can also cause baldness. An early sign of the former is thinning in the eyebrows.

The most common viral infection that causes hair loss is herpes zoster. The first sign is pain and tenderness on the affected area of the scalp, followed by blisters along a nerve line, then localized hair loss. This may result in scarring of the hair follicles, which can lead to permanent hair loss. But antiviral drugs like acyclovir can control the problem. Fungal diseases such as ringworm, though rare in developed countries like the United States, can also cause hair loss. So be alert to any unusual or sudden hair loss and pay an immediate visit to your dermatologist for the correct diagnosis.

MYTHS AND MISDIAGNOSES

To my frustration, hair loss remains a poorly understood area of medicine. We are only just beginning to sift the truth from the myths about its various causes. One of the most popular misconceptions that many doctors still cling to is the notion that hair loss can be caused by stress. In my humble opinion, that is an oversimplification. When hair falls out there is always some physiological cause, and the danger of dismissing hair loss symptoms as something emotional is that a serious underlying condition may be overlooked that will prolong unnecessary hair loss. Yes, stress can exacerbate the symptoms, but it is not the underlying cause. Unconscious hair pulling may be a result of stress, and overstyling hair can also cause it to break or fall out. Always avoid pulling on hair or using styling tools that can dry out the hair shaft or cause excessive traction. Sure, emotional stress doesn't help if you already have a condition, but it does not lead to the kind of diffuse hair loss that would be a concern.

Another common myth surrounding hereditary hair loss is that it is related to an insufficient blood supply to the scalp. So don't bother with a head massage because you think it will help your hair grow. Clogged follicles, a poor diet, a vitamin deficiency, or increased levels of toxins also do not trigger hair loss. Don't let the snake-oil salesmen fool you. And no, you can't shampoo your hair too often or too vigorously! That's just another crazy myth.

There is a lot of misinformation out there, and many people will try to sell you a solution that has no basis in scientific fact. But there are reliable sources with accurate answers about what is going on with your hair and where you can find the best treatments. The following organizations have credible information on their websites:

- The American Academy of Dermatology (www.aad.org)

- The International Society of Hair Restoration Surgery (www.ishrs.org)

- The National Alopecia Areata Foundation (www.naaf.org)

- The American Hair Loss Council (www.ahlc.org)

These are the most common and trustworthy information sources that patients can access for help and support in dealing with their hirsute problems. Hopefully, hair health awareness will grow over the next few years, and your local family practitioner will be able to identify the condition and refer you to the proper specialist before you lose too much of your crowning glory.

WHAT WORKS NOW

Now that we know the underlying causes and where best to find the correct diagnoses, let me bring you up to speed on the latest cutting-edge methods for restoring and maintaining those lush locks of yours.

For women just beginning to notice hair loss and thinning that is not as sudden and severe as some of the conditions described previously, the initial course of treatment is topical. The first thing a woman can do if she is starting to see more scalp than hair is to go to the local pharmacy and pick up an over-the-counter treatment with 2 percent minoxidil, a clear and colorless solution that is usually sold under the brand name Rogaine, although generic versions are also available. Use it twice a day, applying it to the offending areas with a medicine dropper, and be patient for 6 to 12 months to see if it has an effect. Studies show that in most patient groups, 25 percent grow visible hair and 50 percent see less shedding, although the other 25 percent see no effect.[15]

For women who are in the early stages of hair loss, I usually prescribe an agent called spironolactone, which blocks the androgen hormones that can play a role in hair loss and inhibits the receptors where androgens act. Spironolactone is actually a type of water pill, and it's been proven effective in decreasing the amount of hormone activity in women. We usually see a positive effect in the form of hair regrowth within 3 to 6 months of starting treatment. But because spironolactone is a water pill, patients are at risk for losing potassium, so it's necessary to monitor electrolytes at least at 3-month intervals. The drug can also occasionally cause breast tenderness, and in women who are premenopausal, I usually prescribe hormone replacement therapies to try to counteract some of these effects.

In general, estrogen-dominant birth control pills can help prevent further thinning. They don't necessarily produce sufficient regrowth, but a small percentage of women will notice an improvement in their hair loss. The trick is to avoid going on and off any type of hormone replacement, even birth control pills, because it causes hair to go into resting mode and fall out in greater quantities. It's all about avoiding ups and downs and staying in that middle zone to maintain healthy hair.

Another more aggressive approach to regrow hair is to use the prescription-strength topicals and shampoos I custom-blend for my patients. The shampoos are protein based with a sulfosalicylic acid solution to coat the hair shaft, cleanse bacteria and debris, and decrease inflammation of the hair follicle. I usually combine minoxodil (5 percent) with Propecia (finasteride), which inhibits dihydrotestosterone (DHT), a substance in the scalp that can shrink hair follicles. I also use a steroidal anti-inflammatory. We've recently learned that inflammation is a precursor to hair loss, so treating the inflammation early enough can stop it in its tracks. I also like Avodart, the brand name for the drug dutasteride. Avodart was originally approved by the FDA for treatment of benign enlarged prostates, but it was recently approved by the FDA for treatment of hair loss in men and women. It's more effective than Propecia because it reduces the two enzymes responsible for converting testosterone to DHT. Propecia acts on only one of these enyzmes. Dutasteride's dual inhibition has been found to decrease levels of DHT by 90 percent at 2 weeks and 93 percent at 2 years.[16] And yes, even though it was originally a prostate drug for men, Avodart is safe for women in the therapeutic doses necessary for hair restoration. The FDA put it through rigorous clinical testing before approving it for off-label hair loss use.

We've had consistent success with these topicals and shampoos, which, when used alongside high-intensity red light therapy treatments of the scalp, can do wonders in halting and even reversing hair loss. This is an exciting new frontier that is now wide-open to patients. Red light LEDs can stimulate some degree of hair growth by increasing the blood supply to hair follicles.

Laser light is in the visible red light spectrum and is generated through a laser diode. The Revage laser that we use in our practice emits 670 nanometers of visible red light, a level far below that of laser beams that cut or burn tissue. Its heat penetrates tissue to a depth of about 8 to 10 millimeters, so the entire hair organ will be covered to a depth just beyond the hair bulb. The result is drastically reduced inflammation—the precursor to hair loss. Recent studies carried out in my practice show that more than 90 percent of men and women achieve some positive results and more than 44 percent of users see noticeable improvements from the use of red light within the first 6 weeks. Another 45 percent see results within 6 to 12 weeks, and about 55 percent see improvement after 12 weeks.

At our own hair research center, our laser diode machines are going all day. Patients come to us in the early stages of hair loss, often presenting symptoms of burning and itching on the scalp. We do a biopsy to confirm that the cause is inflammation and not some other skin condition. Then

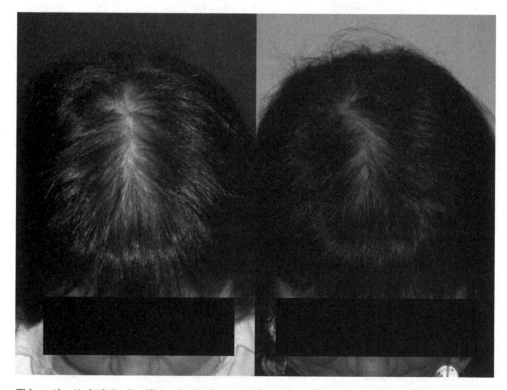

This patient's hair is significantly thicker after being treated with red light LED technology.

patients visit our clinic once a week for 8 weeks for the laser treatment. It takes commitment, but so far the overwhelming majority—about 90 percent—of our hundreds of patients who are participating in this study have expressed great satisfaction with the results, and that is a rare thing in any clinical program. We've seen no side effects, and men and women are able to hang on to what hair they do have, which may be a more than adequate amount if they catch the problem early enough. Many go on to experience new growth with our biostimulating shampoos and topicals, so they can walk away with a head of hair that's almost as thick and healthy as it was in their youth.

RESTORE AND RENEW

When it's too late, and bald or nearly bald patches are already starting to appear at or behind the hairline, it's time for more drastic treatment. Hair transplants have gotten a bad reputation and, until recently, deservedly so. In the procedure, surgeons take follicles from the back and sides of the head, which tend to be immune to pattern baldness, and move them to the front and crown of the head. The success or failure of the procedure depends on how much hair the patient has left to transplant. The older treatments left patients with the obvious rows of hair tufts called plugs that I am stuck with now. If I knew then what I know now, I would have waited, because today's transplant treatments are far more advanced, and the effects look completely natural. With these new microscopic grafting methods, no one could ever tell it's not your natural hairline.

Women are coming in more and more for mini–hair grafts. In fact, almost half of my hair transplant patients are females in their forties and fifties. Many have an area right behind their hairline where as much as 90 percent of the hair is gone, but they still have a decent quantity of hair in the very back of their head, which makes them great transplant candidates. Unlike most balding men, women have a viable hairline, and what they need most is dense hair growth behind it. To achieve this, I use a new technique called slit grafting where I remove very small slits of scalp for transplantation. This has revolutionized the process of hair restoration surgery in women. Because the grafts are so fine, there is little scarring at the back of the head where the hair is harvested, and there is no cosmetic deficit. You can barely notice after the procedure that you've actually had a hair transplant. The hair just begins to grow naturally, and it is impossible to detect unless you take a magnifying glass to the back of the head to search for scars.

Follicular unit extractions, or minigrafts, are recently developed transplant techniques that allow surgeons to use the smallest possible recipient sites for the greatest amount of hair density, and they have the least amount of downtime. Patients can usually opt for in-office procedures with a local anesthetic or twilight sedation if they prefer. But these techniques are for candidates who require only a modest change in hair fullness, and donor areas on the back of the head need to be thick. Hair color, texture, waviness, and curl can also affect cosmetic outcomes. Sometimes surgeons will use a combination of grafting techniques for best outcomes.

Check out as many before and after pictures of hair transplant patients as you can. It's an exacting and painstaking cosmetic procedure, so the same rules apply for choosing a skillful and safe doctor. Also note that many hair restoration centers advertise heavily and try to take advantage of desperate people. The better ones, however, offer to replace any transplants that do not take. When you interview doctors, find out what kinds of results they promise, their success rate, how many types of procedures they perform, and how many years they have been doing transplants.

One promising new and incision-free hair transplant method that works for patients looking for both modest and dramatic change is an automated version of follicular unit extraction (FUE), which uses specially designed punches that are just under a millimeter in size. Called NeoGraft, this new FUE technology can harvest and transplant as many as 3,000 grafts over 2 days. It is arguably the most precise and natural-looking hair transplant available, as well as the least traumatic and invasive for patients. In the past, FUE grafts were extremely labor-intensive when done correctly because hair follicles had to be separated manually, and few doctors offered them because of the degree of difficulty. There was also a risk of losing grafts in the long and painstaking transplantation process.

Not so now. The new FUE method uses a motorized punch that gently rotates around each individual graft in perfectly cylindrical shapes. It then employs a controlled and gentle suction to slide out the follicles smoothly and uniformly, so there is no pulling and twisting as with forceps. The strength of the suction can be adjusted to accommodate different skin types and the various punch sizes. The grafts are then collected in a small canister that gently and frequently mists grafts with sterile saline to keep them moist during the harvesting process until they are ready for implantation. The transplant sites are tailored to the exact length of the harvested grafts and inserted with gentle pneumatic pressure so that the grafts are implanted to the exact depth, leaving a smooth, level recipient surface and preventing any ingrown or exposed follicles. After the grafts have been separated from the canister, they are withdrawn, or autoloaded, into an implantation cannula

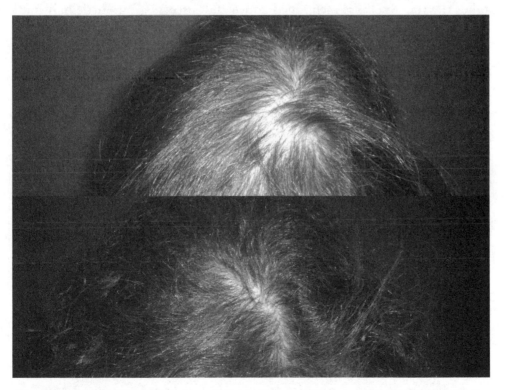

This patient opted for a follicular unit transplant and now has a full, thick head of hair.

using negative pneumatic pressure. Once they are in the cannula, the follicles are inserted into the recipient site using positive pneumatic pressure. Though there remains a concern that some hairs may be destroyed in the graft, Neo-Graft is a promising technique that eliminates much of the guesswork.

NeoGraft solves two of the key challenges to hair transplants:

First, it eliminates or mostly eliminates the scar on the back of the head. Traditionally, a hair transplant procedure requires the doctor to take a flap from the back of the head to use for donor hair. Unlike the minigrafts described earlier, more dramatic transplants require much larger grafts of skin tissue. But NeoGraft punches out follicles so they are ready for reimplantation, leaving tiny holes on the donor site that will close over and become invisible over time.

Second, the NeoGraft eliminates much of the extensive cutting and prep work associated with a hair transplant. In a traditional transplant, the doctor takes the flap or ellipse mentioned above and dissects it into little hair units for implantation. Because the NeoGraft machine harvests the hair in a way that makes it ready for reimplantation, this step is basically removed. From a patient's perspective, the reduced scar is the most significant improvement. But anything that lessens the painstaking preparation and cutting a doctor will have to perform will eventually help reduce the price of this procedure, which can cost as much as $20,000 depending on how many grafts the patient needs. And the cosmetic effect of NeoGraft is much more natural because of the tiny individual follicle plantations. So for men in particular who fear that obvious hairline, NeoGraft is a great option.

BUMPER CROP

Until we have the next-generation solution for hair loss, transplants and topical treatments are the best options we have. But there are a few exciting new possibilities on the hair horizon, from stem cell stimulation to gene therapy and tissue engineering, also known as hair cloning. There's plenty of incentive for companies to stay on this quest for the holy grail of hair growth. In the United States alone, consumers spend more than $1 billion a year on hair treatments and transplants. Now that restrictions on scientific research on stem cells have been lifted somewhat, the race for that magic bullet is on as dozens of biotech companies and university labs study ways to stimulate the growth of new hair follicles. Some viable solutions may be just a few years away. Others may not happen in my lifetime. But early signs are promising.

Top physicians are already experimenting with combinations of hair transplants and PRP—the platelet-rich plasma therapy I discussed in Chapter 8. They're injecting patients' scalps with their own blood plasma, which is rich in growth factors. It's like fertilizing the field for a bumper crop after you've planted the seedlings. In theory, the hair grafts themselves will grow in thicker and healthier and provide more coverage. We're starting to use growth factors together with transplants in our own practice and seeing excellent results, although we need to do more research to determine how much of the improvement is due to PRP.

A study at the University of Pennsylvania that generated a lot of media buzz 3 years ago found that a combination of wounding the skin on the scalps of mice and treating the wounds with various growth factors and biostimulants could help produce new hair follicles, challenging the long-held belief that once a hair follicle is dead, it never comes back.[17] This breakthrough led to the creation of a biotech company called Follica, which is testing methods to help reproduce the regenerative powers of wound healing for human hair. Follica uses a form of microdermabrasion to induce mild injury to the scalp, scrape off dead skin cells, and promote repair by deeper cells. But it's not yet known how long this new hair will last or how safe the procedure is. The research is still years away from being implemented in the real world of a dermatologist's practice.

Another company, Aderans Research Institute, is using tissue engineering to try to reproduce new hair follicles. They are taking two types of cells from the scalp and growing them in culture in the hope that they will "signal" to each other to promote the creation of follicles. Those cultured cells are then injected back into the scalp to create what are essentially "hair seeds" intended to grow into hair follicles. Although this is commonly referred to as hair cloning, no follicles are actually created in the culture. It's up to the recipient's own body to take over and make that happen. Numerous other companies around the world are also exploring this concept.

Probably one of the most exciting new developments in hair regeneration, and the closest to becoming available in the marketplace, comes out of a company based in California called Histogen. In the interest of full disclosure, I have just joined Histogen's scientific advisory board and will be involved in the next stage of clinical trials for their own hair regrowth applications.

Histogen is a regenerative medicine company that was launched in 2007 to develop stem cell solutions for skin and hair. Inside its specially designed bioreactors, Histogen has been able to re-create embryonic conditions to grow stem cells from the fibroblasts of newborn foreskins. No animal or embryonic stem cells are used in any of their products, but the result is a cocktail of embryonic-like proteins and growth factors that can be turned into numerous products, including hair follicle and skin cell tissue. The company just completed a year-long double-blind, placebo-controlled clinical pilot study of its Hair Stimulating Complex (HSC), using 24 patients. The result after a single treatment was an increase in the number of new hairs, increased hair density, and rapid hair growth that has continued over a 12-month period in each patient. In the realm of hair restoration, this is a phenomenal discovery.[18]

I'll be involved in the next round of clinical trials that will be examining the safety and efficacy of HSC as an injectable for hair growth. We'll be determining protocols such as optimum treatment dosage and delivery. Of all these extraordinary and groundbreaking developments in hair restoration science, this may bring us the closest yet to that ultimate goal of new hair follicle generation. When HSC hits the market, probably within the next 5 years, the impact on millions of people suffering from permanent hair loss will be huge.

Believe me, I know what it's like to see more and more strands of hair on your comb or watch them circle down the bathtub drain. I've been there. But don't despair. Research in this field has come a long way, and so have the treatments. We're making it our business to learn what truly causes hair loss so that we can prevent it as well as treat it. Scientific breakthroughs are happening every year. What's happening in South Korea and Japan in this field, particularly surrounding the treatment of hair loss with stem cells and cloning, is extraordinary, and our own scientists are joining the rest of the world in the race to do what everyone once thought was impossible—cure baldness.

Meanwhile, you don't have to grow bald gracefully. There's plenty you can do today to stop hair loss in its tracks and keep those locks looking luscious for years to come.

CHAPTER FIFTEEN

THE NEW FRONTIER

THE FUTURISTIC FIGHT AGAINST FLAB

Everywhere you turn in the quest for naturalistic youth and beauty, there's an exciting new frontier that seems like pure science fiction, and our relentless fight against body fat is no exception.

One of my patients, Janet, came to me 6 months after giving birth, complaining that even with diet and exercise, she was struggling to drop that extra 20 pounds of post-baby weight. Somehow, the fat in her body had redistributed and was concentrated in the lower half of her torso. She was left with a pair of love handles that spilled over the top of her jeans like muffin tops and made her self-conscious. But except for that area and a small but pronounced pooch in her lower abdomen, she was in pretty good shape.

Janet was dead set against surgery. For her, even a minor liposuction procedure was out of the question because it involved a small incision, and she would do anything but cut the skin. So instead she opted for Zeltiq Coolsculpting, a new non-invasive procedure based on cryolipolysis, a technology that uses extreme cold to target and destroy fat cells. The device, which was approved by the FDA for fat reduction in 2009, is pressed against the body part to be treated, targeting the fat cells in that area with extreme cold without damaging surrounding cells. This action spurs an inflammatory response within the body, which causes it to naturally dispose of the damaged fat cells. Zeltiq is virtually painless, and it usually requires only one treatment, although some patients may need a follow-up 4 months later when the full results have had a chance to kick in. But, as we warned Janet, the results would not be dramatic. Nonsurgical body contouring is not for removing large amounts of fat; it's more for patients who wish to treat localized problem areas, such as a small tummy pooch or love handles. Some overall circumference reduction and a smoother contour were about as much as we could lead her to expect. She would not turn into Heidi Klum overnight.

"It's okay, Doc, I get it," said Janet. "I'll keep up with the training, but I just want to get to another level. I'm sick of wearing Spanx every time I go out!"

We targeted Janet's problem areas: her tummy, her love handles, some pockets of fat on her inner thighs, and the jiggle on her upper arms. During the procedure, her tissue was drawn into a cup with mild vacuum pressure. No anesthesia was required. Janet did experience some mild discomfort with the initial cold contact as the procedure began, but the slight pain went away after about 10 minutes.

Several days after her procedure, the cooled fat cells began to shrink through a process called apoptosis. This continued for several months as the damaged fat cells were slowly digested and expelled from her body.

By the time Janet came back for a follow-up visit 4 months later, she'd lost 2 inches off her midsection and the love handles had virtually disappeared, all without the pain and risk of surgical incisions and with no downtime. She was thrilled because she saw improvement in the stubborn areas around her midsection she hadn't been able to budge the old-fashioned way. Now she could fit into a pair of jeans two sizes smaller and didn't need an extra treatment. Her expectations were realistic and she got the result she wanted. In short, she was the ideal Zeltiq patient.

ABS TO ENVY

I've always done my best to stay in shape. And at age 40, I was doing pretty well. I know everybody thinks they look younger than their years, but I can honestly say that a lifetime of exercise, clean living, and taking supplements has helped me maintain a youthful appearance. But still . . . I'm 40. And there are certain changes in body shape that are inevitable.

It got to the point where no matter how cleanly I ate and no matter how many sit-ups and crunches and leg lifts I did, I still had those dreaded love handles. They say they're the last to go, but in my case they were hanging on for dear life. Even at 165 pounds and 10 percent body fat! You can't fight genetics, I guess.

I know it's a common complaint. Humans aren't really designed to look like perfect physical specimens. We're designed to survive, and that requires having a storage of fat in case of famine—which may not exist in the typical American lifestyle, but our bodies haven't caught up to our contemporary conditions. Women have that "extra" on their hips, men have it on their obliques. And I wanted it gone. Having it sucked out surgically seemed like the only answer.

After doing considerable research, I went to see Dr. Sadick about some liposuction. I was prepared for the pain, but I was a little leery about going under general anesthesia. The good doc filled me in about a relatively new procedure—laser lipolysis. At first I assumed it was just a fancy term for the same old thing; after all, the only way to get the fat out is to go in and get it, right? But this laser lipo was not only less invasive, it required little more than a mild sedative. I was informed that in less than an hour, my love handles would be gone. Well, at least after the swelling subsided. So I made the appointment.

The procedure was as easy as I was told it would be. After popping a couple of lorazepam, I relaxed for a while until I was comfortably buzzed. I reclined on the patient chair for a shot of something to provide a little local numbing via an IV tube— something called tumescent anesthesia. We waited for about half an hour for it to take effect. Then the doctor and his assistant went to work.

I didn't feel a thing the entire time and was even chatting with the doc and his team

Welcome to the future. Some of the most exciting advances in nonsurgical cosmetic enhancement are for treating localized fat deposits and cellulite all over the body. Today it is actually possible to eliminate small areas of fat by freezing it or sonically eradicating the adipose tissue. No throughout the procedure. It was hard to believe that a laser fiber inserted under my skin was heating and melting the fat layering my obliques. Once it was over I assumed I was going to get a few stitches, but the incision was so small there was no need. It looked like two tiny cuts on each side of my waist. All that was required were a couple of Band-Aids.

I was told to expect some soreness that night and was given a prescription for a painkiller, but I didn't even need it. Being an avid exercise enthusiast, I'm used to a little soreness. The only inconvenience was that I needed to wear a compression garment for a few days to restrict swelling. It also sucked that I couldn't exercise for a week. But other than that, the post-op downtime was little more than a few hours. I could go about my day, albeit gingerly.

When I first removed the garment, I must admit it didn't seem like there was much of a difference, but Dr. Sadick assured me that was the result of residual swelling and it would subside in a few days. He was right! A week after the surgery, the results were phenomenal. My torso had the best "V" taper I've seen since my twenties.

It was at my follow-up visit that I asked about skin looseness. I knew a few people who'd had lipo and their skin never quite sprang back after being stretched out from all the extra fat for so many years. This was where laser lipo makes such a big difference. The technique stimulates collagen formation so that the skin gets tighter and firmer as time goes by. How cool is that?

Call me vain, but every day it's a great feeling to look into the mirror and like what I see. Now I can appreciate the results of my work in the gym without it being ruined by that stubborn flab on my sides. There aren't even any noticeable scars. It would be impossible to tell anything was done. The picture is complete. It's been 6 months since my procedure, and I am loving it! I'm actually more motivated to work out because I know now there's no excuse not to be in the best shape of my life. But I couldn't have done it had I not taken that last step. It wasn't cheap; it cost more than $5,000. But I don't regret it for a second.

Greg C.

cutting. No liposuction. Just non-invasive technology like LipoSonix, which uses high-intensity focused ultrasound to reduce unwanted fat. My research group is even experimenting with acoustic wave therapy to blast off cellulite.

Many of these non-invasive fat removal options are just months away from FDA approval. These treatments are not for obese patients, but for average people with problem areas they might otherwise turn to surgery to treat. These alternatives are much safer than traditional surgery. Anytime you penetrate the skin there are risks, and patients can spend hours under the knife—circumstances under which most anesthesia-related deaths occur. This new technology has the potential to gradually shave inches off those love handles without the risk or the pain and swelling of traditional liposuction.

Make no mistake: Most of these procedures are still in the earliest stages of development and often don't deliver results sufficient to justify their cost. One that has received a lot of hype lately, the Lapex 2000, uses a combination of massage and low-level laser energy to break up fat cells without surgery. It is non-invasive and painless and uses a diode laser to reach deep into the dermis and attack subcutaneous fat. The theory is that Lapex stimulates the fat cells, causing them to release their contents of water, glycerol, and free fatty acids, effectively shrinking them. The free fatty acids are then absorbed into the lymphatic system, and the glycerol goes into the bloodstream and is eventually flushed out the usual way, through urine. Patients are then advised to do a little cardio following their sessions, eat a balanced diet, and drink plenty of water.

But the results of Lapex 2000 are less than impressive, and it's not clear if the weight reduction is from the extra cardio or the technology itself. Zerona is another treatment that has been receiving a lot of buzz. It's similar to Lapex in that it uses low-energy cold laser therapy externally for spot fat reduction. If it is to be believed, a recent study published in *Cosmetic Surgery Times* showed an average 1.08-inch reduction over six treatments using Zerona.[19] But the therapy also includes lymphatic massage and vitamin supplements. Both work to some degree, but the question is how and for how long? Is the treatment cost-effective given the degree of efficacy? And what are the best protocols?

Yet the menu of options for body contouring is substantial and growing. Lapex and Zerona are at the lower end of the non-invasive body-contouring spectrum and are better suited for smaller areas of the body. They are also the least expensive of the nonsurgical body-contouring devices, costing between $150 and $400 per treatment, depending on your geography. But you get what you pay for.

FROM JUST OKAY
TO PRETTY GOOD

More technology is constantly becoming available, and many of the machines I now view with healthy skepticism may soon have advanced two or three more generations, with enough proven results for efficacy and safety. But for now, here's a list of what is available today, along with my honest appraisal in ascending order of price and results:

• **Arasys Inch-Loss System**—A muscle-stimulating machine that claims to give you a workout without the exertion. It was originally created for muscle-wasting conditions and mimics an intense form of isometric exercise, except that instead of exerting themselves, patients lie on a table hooked up to eight wires that are attached to a control box with eight dials. Nerve endings around the patient's muscles are affected by contact with faradic waveforms—a series of short pulses a few milliseconds in length—which subsequently cause the muscles to contract. The manufacturer say it takes about 10 sessions to see results. Patients say at the end of the session that it feels as if their muscles have had a workout, although the procedure is not painful. Proponents of the technology say that a 20-minute Arasys session can have the same body-sculpting impact as 300 sit-ups. Perhaps, although there is not a lot of science to back up this claim. It costs $150 to $300 per treatment.

• **Cynosure's Cellulaze**—A minimally invasive surgical approach to attacking cellulite beneath the surface of the skin. It uses laser technology to target the depressions and fat deposits beneath the skin's surface that form cellulite. Under local anesthesia, the physician inserts a small cannula, which generates controlled heat to break up and release no tension from connective tissue. Approved for use in Europe, where patient results have been positive, this looks like a promising long-term solution for cellulite.

• **VelaShape and SmoothShapes**—These devices are used more for cellulite, but it is also possible to lose inches with them. Both rely on a combination of laser technology, suction, and massage. We have found the results for both machines are good but not great. They are certainly a step up from the endermology offered at so-called medi-spas (where someone with a medical background is nowhere to be seen). Endermology uses massage and suction, but not the laser technology, and can produce a slight (if temporary) improvement in the appearance of cellulite. VelaShape looks like a giant industrial vacuum, which is appropriate, because a large handpiece suctions the body while specially designed rollers massage the tissue to increase blood flow. The SmoothShapes handpiece looks a little sleeker, but it combines the same elements of laser energy with mechanical massage and suction. Neither treatment is painful, and if you enjoy a vigorous body rub, you may even find it pleasant. Both cost between $1,000 and $3,000 for a full series of treatments. Both treatments are more suited to fine contouring than to major debulking. They may be good add-ons for patients who have had liposuction or lost a significant amount of weight the old-fashioned way, because they can help tighten and tone loose skin and smooth out the lumps and bumps caused by adhesions.

• **Accent XL**—Arguably the next level in efficacy, Accent harnesses radiofrequency energy at two levels. Again, the system consists of handpieces attached to a large mounted monitor with control settings that is the source of power. A treatment may last approximately half an hour and is generally painless. The session involves the use of two handpieces that resemble futuristic toy guns. They are passed over the area of the body you are looking to improve. The skin may feel some warm sensation, but the Accent utilizes a cooling technique to minimize any pain. One handpiece is bipolar—for dermal heating to help tighten the tissue closer to the skin's surface. The second handpiece, the unipolar device, reaches deeper below the dermis for fat and cellulite reduction. Some practitioners recommend it as a treatment to tighten the skin prior to liposuction procedures and to smooth out the skin after the lipo treatment, marketing it as a less costly version of Thermage. It doesn't have the disposable tips used in Thermage and costs about $300 per treatment, depending on the size of the area to be treated. But it takes several treatments to see results.

• **Thermage**—Whether for face tightening or body contouring, Thermage is the gold standard. It's more expensive than Accent, costing about $2,500 per treatment, but it's also much more powerful than the other tighteners, it requires only one session, and the results can last up to 2 years. We've seen pretty dramatic results from Thermage use in large areas of the body that need tightening and toning, including the abdomen, thighs, and buttocks. There's also some evidence that the deep-heating energy destroys fat cells. A handheld device delivers the energy, which comes from a boxy computer-controlled monitor mounted on wheels with control settings for temperature. The doctor will apply a numbered grid to the area to be treated, to map out where the heat should be applied. In the latest generation of the machine, a Therma-Cool system delivers a controlled amount of energy through the treatment tip. With each touch to the skin, the ThermaTip device, which resembles an oversize electric toothbrush without the brush, uniformly heats a volume of collagen in the deeper layers of the skin and its underlying tissue while simultaneously helping to protect the outer layer of the skin with cooling. Patients will experience a brief spike of heat that's tolerable, and the doctor will adjust the heat according to patient feedback to assure maximum results with the least amount of discomfort. Patients are sometimes given painkillers ahead of the treatment. The good news is that the procedure is over within about 45 minutes and repeat treatments are not necessary. One Thermage session will last you about a year.

• **Zeltiq**—The treatment we used on Janet is one of the potentially more exciting technological advances in non-ablative body contouring that essentially freezes away the fat. During the procedure, the selected area is drawn up between two cooling plates and held in place by suction. This handpiece also looks like a vacuum accessory, and it is attached by a hose to an upright mobile device. The procedures takes 1 hour per area, so if you want both love handles treated, think 2 hours. If you also want your abdomen treated, think up to 4 hours, depending on your size. Because fat cells are more sensitive to cold, the precise temperature maintenance during the procedure begins to disrupt fat cells without damaging other layers of the skin. Immediately after the treatment, the treated skin sticks up for a few seconds like a frozen cone before it settles back into place. Patients may experience redness on the area, like a giant hickey, and occasionally some numbness or tingling for a day or two. It takes a couple of months to notice the results, which are not drastic but definitely noticeable. Testing has shown no increase in blood lipids or blood cholesterol. Some other procedures that "melt fat" have concerned physicians who fear that the body cannot properly process the large quantity of fat suddenly introduced into the lymphatic system. Zeltiq appears to override this concern as it takes several weeks for the fat to be expelled. The problem is more one of delivery than outcome: The procedure is not exactly comfortable, and it is a long time to ask a patient to sit still under those circumstances. And it's not cheap: It costs about $3,000 for the three to four treatment cycles. (One area costs about $750.)

• **UltraShape**—Uses focused ultrasound to disrupt the fat cells and break them down so they can be metabolized by the body. The system's space age monitor and power source looks like a robotic character out of a *Star Wars* movie, with a circular transducer attachment that passes over the area to be treated. The principle behind the UltraShape treatment is to harness the energy so that the ultrasound waves do not injure the surrounding tissue of blood vessels. A transducer concentrates the ultrasound waves to the layer of subcutaneous fat just below the dermis. Various clinical studies in the United States and overseas have noted positive results in body contouring, with up to 2.5 inches lost after three to four sessions. However, there needs to be more testing. I am not yet fully convinced of the safety of the procedure. Results of Phase III clinical testing are positive, but I want to see more proven protocols. Ultrasound energy produces a mechanical pressure wave through soft tissue, which is safe for diagnostic sonography testing (viewing a fetus, for example) because it uses such low levels of energy. But once you start upping the frequency, it's not clear how well that energy is controlled by the practitioner. For years, ultrasound has been used medically to reach and treat clear targets like tumors, fibroids, and kidney stones, but the application for cosmetic fat removal is still in relative infancy, with many questions remaining about best practices. What is the appropriate depth? What is the risk of the energy reflecting off bone and causing intense pain or surface burns? How do you individualize the energy levels for each patient? Because it is not yet widely available here, it's also hard to gauge an average cost, but patients who have had this procedure overseas have reported that it cost between $3,000 and $9,000 for treatments before they saw satisfactory results.

• **UltraShape Contour I Ver3**—The next generation of UltraShape uses a combination of focused ultrasound and radiofrequency to break up deeper layers of fat. It looks like its space age predecessor with the addition of a handheld device that combines radiofrequency energy with suction, to pretreat the fat and dissolve microbubbles in the skin tissue before the ultrasound is applied, for a smoother, more uniform result. The handpiece is used again after the ultrasound energy is applied to increase circulation to tighten the tissue and speed up the process of fat clearance. I expect we'll see more of these combined technologies in the future.

• **LipoSonix**—Also uses ultrasonic energy to disrupt fatty tissue and is in the final phase of clinical testing by the FDA, although it's been approved in Canada, where a treatment package costs about $4,000. Like UltraShape, LipoSonix is intended to treat small areas of stubborn fat in the thigh, buttock, abdomen, and back regions that are resistant to diet and exercise. According to the machine's developers, this procedure can be effective at destroying excess fat at depths of an inch or more without doing any damage to the epidermis. A decrease in cellulite may accompany an overall reduction in fat. Again, the machine is a large, upright mobile device, with an armlike attachment complete with a tracking monitor that produces ultrasound images of where the energy is going and a bulky piece with two handles on each side that delivers the energy. The main difference between UltraShape and Lipo-Sonix is the delivery method. LipoSonix produces more thermal than focused energy and may be more painful. It's a very promising technology, but again, there needs to be more testing for safety and efficacy. Doctors in the United States have not had the opportunity to test the focused ultrasound machine themselves, because the machines will not be available here until they receive FDA approval. Sometimes we get to use technology off-label, before it receives FDA approval for a designated treatment. Even though it was only recently approved for body contouring, Zeltiq, for example, has been used here for 2 years because it had been previously approved for use as an anesthetic for certain skin treatments. But that's not the case with every new technology.

I believe the gold standard of nonsurgical, painless, effective body contouring is just a couple of years away. But even now we have a cornucopia of treatments for every type of body problem, from skin laxity to excess fat and cellulite, and patients can already look forward to achieving smoother skin, slimmer contours, and a more toned appearance with much less pain and downtime than we ever thought possible.

This is only the beginning. Sheer demand from patients will propel the science and technology forward to a point where it's cost-effective and completely safe. Since 2000, liposuction was consistently among the top five plastic surgery procedures, according to the American Society of Plastic Surgeons (ASPS).[20] In 2009, 283,735 Americans had a liposuction procedure, according to the American Society for Aesthetic Plastic Surgery.[21] The number of people seeking body-contouring procedures will surely explode once safe, simple, and relatively painless non-invasive technology becomes more widely available.

But we still have a long way to go. For now, most of the technology previously described is not widely available in the United States, and when it is, practitioners are using it off-label for cosmetic use. There need to be more patient studies and more evidence of significant improvement and patient satisfaction before I wholeheartedly endorse any of these procedures. For now, I am keeping a close eye on every new development and making sure I can get my hands on as many of these new machines as possible.

SUCK IT UP

Meanwhile, I tell most of my patients who want to remove stubborn areas of fat to stick to liposuction. That's right. For once in this book I am saying surgery is the better option for most, albeit a surgical procedure of the minimally invasive kind. Liposuction has seen many advances beyond the traditional, mechanical force of fat extraction that make it safer and more effective, with less bruising, swelling, pain, and downtime. Lipo can remove much larger amounts of adipose tissue, and with certain procedures, there's the added benefit of skin tightening as the area heals.

Despite its overwhelming popularity, many patients still fear liposuction. They've seen the starlets with the lumpy torsos caused by uneven procedures, and they've heard the media reports of patients undergoing large-scale debulking and dying on the table or having serious postsurgical complications. Well, yes, there are always risks when you go under anesthesia for a considerable length of time. And results vary depending on the skill level of the practitioner. Like any medical procedure, this is not something to jump into without doing some serious research first. Before you opt for any form of liposuction, ask your prospective surgeon the following questions:

- What is your experience with lipo/body contouring, and how many procedures do you perform per year?

- Which technology or specific lipo procedure will give me the best results, and why?

- How much skin tightening can I expect from laser lipo?

- What kind of swelling and drainage issues should I expect?

- How long is the surgery, and what is the recovery period/downtime?

- What are the immediate effects post-op?

- What postsurgical care will I require?

- How long does it take before I can see results?

- Is one type of procedure better than another for a particular area of my body?

- Can I see before and after pictures?

- What other results should I expect from the procedure?

- How much weight can I expect to safely lose?

- Will smoking affect my healing time and results? (Your surgeon should answer, "Yes!")

Your doctor's willingness to answer and provide you with all the information you request will speak volumes. Meanwhile, you should educate yourself about what's most current in liposuction. Besides traditional liposuction, which involves the vacuum-assisted removal of subcutaneous fat via a hollow metal cannula, there are three other kinds of lipolysis: tumescent, ultrasound, and laser-assisted:

• **Tumescent Liposuction**—Uses a diluted cocktail of local anesthetic and other medications, which are injected into the fat layers prior to lipolysis. This causes the skin tissue to become swollen and rigid, making it easier for the surgeon to control where he or she is penetrating during the procedure. The numbing effects of these medications mean the patient does not require general anesthesia, so the process is much safer than traditional lipo. The physician can remove more fat at different levels beneath the skin and even ask the patient to shift position to allow better access to the areas to be treated. It requires no hospital stay, and there are fewer side effects such as bleeding and bruising.

• **Ultrasound-Assisted Lipoplasty**—Uses sound waves internally to break down fat cells. An ultrasound cannula with a sound-emitting mechanism is injected to loosen the fat, which is then extracted with a second, hollow cannula. The ultrasound is essentially a pretreatment for the actual liposuction. By contrast, traditional lipo relies on the brute force of the physician to mechanically break up the fat with a larger, much scarier-looking cannula, which is used in a crisscross motion, or on power-assisted lipo, which vibrates the cannula to break up the fat. With ultrasound, there is some pain and heating from sound waves, but again there is much less trauma compared with traditional lipo because the fat is broken down to a much thinner consistency, which makes for easier extraction with smaller incisions. Because sound wave energy is so powerful, it's also effective at breaking up particularly stubborn, fibrous pockets of fat. Patients are usually awake for this procedure, and it can be done on an outpatient basis.

• **Laser-Assisted Lipoplasty**—The latest and most promising advance in the evolution of body sculpting. The two makers of this type of liposuction technology are SmartLipo, which came out with it first, and SmoothLipo, although there is little difference between the two. It is also a pretreatment, using a series of laser fibers inserted through microcannulas of varying length and diameter to heat and liquefy the adipose cells. This is then followed by traditional liposuction to remove the fat. Because the fat is in liquid form, the cannula tube used to extract it is less than 2 millimeters in diameter and therefore requires a much smaller incision than other forms of liposuction. The result is less bruising, bleeding, swelling, or scarring. Yes, there is a slight risk of thermal injury if the surgeon fails to keep the laser cannula moving, and laser lipo is also better suited to smaller areas of fat. But judicious body contouring and an aesthetic eye can create the appearance of much greater weight loss. As with all of these technologies, the right doctor, not the instrument, is essential to best results. One advantage to the technology is that if you have only one area to treat, you can opt for a local anesthetic. As with tumescent lipo, the surgeon will pump you full of fluid before using the laser, usually a mixture of saline, lidocaine to numb you, and ephedrine to constrict the blood vessels and minimize blood loss. It won't be entirely painless. You'll feel some pinching and pulling. But my patients tell me it's tolerable.

THE BEST, FOR NOW

Personally, I am a fan of laser lipolysis. I recommend it more than any of the other body-contouring procedures. It's extremely effective on localized fat deposits on your stomach, flanks, thighs, buttocks, neck, upper arms, calves, and ankles. It is also much safer than other liposuction procedures. The trauma is minimal. Within a couple of hours, the patient can go back to his or her business. There's some slight swelling, but that subsides after a few days, and it's not necessary for SmartLipo patients to wear a compression bandage for more than a week, although some doctors advise their patients to wear one for 2 weeks. This garment helps reduce postsurgical swelling and prevents the skin from stretching out. There is the significant added benefit of skin tightening, because the heating effect under the skin produces collagen. A recent study has shown that the skin contracts as much as 17 percent, so patients don't have to fear the saggy skin associated with traditional liposuction.[22]

According to some recent findings, laser lipolysis can also decrease cellulite. This is by no means guaranteed, but I have had several female patients

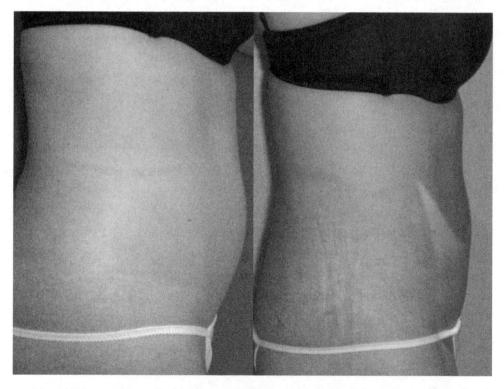

Liposuction and laser liposuction are still the gold standard in body contouring.

who sought treatment for fat and cellulite deposits. I warned them that while I could improve their contour and reduce their overall circumference, cellulite is an entirely different problem (more on cellulite at the end of this chapter). But each time, we were pleasantly surprised. After 6 months—the time it usually takes for the dermis layer of the skin to fully contract, heal, and produce collagen—their cellulite had all but disappeared.

By contrast, traditional lipo can leave the skin less smooth. If patients have skin laxity, they can end up with loose flab in areas where large amounts of fat have been removed. Often, patients look better in clothes but worse without clothes. Excess treatment can result in dimpling and divots, and it's not possible to get every fat cell, so patients can end up with unsightly lumps, particularly if they don't maintain their weight and the fat cells grow. But the more advanced techniques, especially laser lipo, allow for more uniform fat removal, creating a much smoother contour.

THE NEXT LEVEL

Emerging technology is taking lipo a step further with computer-controlled procedures using radiofrequency energy. Proper protocols are being worked out with extensive clinical testing at this very moment, and FDA approval is still pending. But computer-controlled body contouring promises to be one of the safest and most effective procedures yet. Energy is delivered from the lipo suction cannula tip, causing simultaneous melting and removal of fat but also controlled heating of the skin. This heating allows for improved skin tightening. External and internal skin temperature sensors minimize the risk of burns because the energy is instantly switched off by the computer as soon as the optimal level of heating is reached. It's a user-friendly, closed-loop power delivery system that heats subdermal fat safely, quickly, and uniformly. The correlation between heating temperature, length of application of the energy, and degree of skin tightening still has to be worked out. But the science is almost there.

There are also new laser systems that track the heat delivered through laser lipolysis. This is important because it allows the surgeon to "see" inside the body and know exactly where the cannula is and how much heat is being delivered. The added benefit to this new advanced tracking system is significant because it eliminates the potential for overheating, burning, or delivering inconsistent energy. Simply put, there is a lower risk of adhesions, less dependence on the technique, and ultimately better results.

At least 80 percent of the success of these procedures depends on the skill of the surgeon, as well as the candidate for the surgery, not to mention their expectations. If they are holding steady at within 30 pounds of their ideal weight, they can expect good results. However, if a patient is older with poor skin elasticity, for example, too much fat removal will cause the skin to sag. None of these procedures are ideal for the obese, because the more fat removed, the higher the surgical risk. Sure, you can extract more when the patient is unconscious on the operating table, but that's when you run into problems. A conscious patient is always the safer choice. You'd be amazed at how many of my patients actually enjoy being awake during the procedure. Several people who've gone through lipo with a local anesthetic have described a feeling of elation and relief at seeing all that fat coming out of their bodies, particularly when they are debulking their stomach pooches and flanks. One of my patients, Alison, joked it was like watching all those Dunkin' Donuts sprinkles finally leaving her body!

There are no proven internal health benefits to removing fat in this way. It doesn't reduce blood pressure or lower your cholesterol. There was some concern that the lipids released into the body after some of these body-contouring procedures could in fact increase triglyceride counts, but that fear has been laid to rest with extensive clinical research. And at the end of the day, it's always healthier to a have a smaller waist. The less visceral fat surrounding your vital organs, the better.

STICK IT

Another way to get rid of fat has nothing to do with high-tech machines—that is, if you don't mind being a pincushion. While it has not yet been approved by the FDA in the United States, treatments have been performed throughout Europe and South America for over 50 years. The treatment is particularly popular in Hollywood, where residents seek the best mesotherapy specialists with proven track records.

There are two different types of injectable approaches that can reduce localized fat deposits on the hips, abdomen, and buttocks and improve areas of unsightly cellulite. The first relies on a product commonly used in Europe called Lipostabil. Lipostabil is a combination of two active ingredients—sodium deoxycholate and phosphatidylcholine. These two emulsifying agents act as detergents to liquefy fat cells when injected, thus minimizing unwanted bulges. The second mesotherapy approach is the injection of biologically active substances such as aminophylline, isoproterenol, ephedrine, carnitine, and herbal preparations, among others. These combinations dissolve unwanted fat cells with a similar emulsifying action. There have been scientific studies published in the *Journal of Dermatologic Surgery* regarding the use of phosphatidylcholine and deoxycholate, showing a significant clinical effect on destroying fat cells and also in treating benign fatty tumors such as lipomas.[23]

But these are very technique-dependent therapies. Thanks to lack of standardization and improper use, infection, skin ulcerations, skin irregularities, lumpiness, and other complications have been reported. The procedure is commonly employed by physicians who do not traditionally treat aesthetic problems. In an earlier chapter about the dangers of overhyping a treatment, I mentioned lipodissolve, a highly controversial variation on mesotherapy that uses a combination of bile acids and detergents that eat through fat tissue. Many patients were left with skin depressions and painful knots under the injection sites that did not go away, and several medi-spas have been sued by the FDA for promoting the treatment and making false claims. In general, it's the lack of standardization in the ingredients and technique that is the main problem with mesotherapy, but several companies are looking to change that.

We recently completed a successful trial for a California-based drug developer called Lithera that used a combination of steroids and detergents to shrink and dissolve the fat. (Another developer out in California, Kythera Biopharmaceuticals, is also attempting to develop and standardize mesotherapy treatments.) After 8 weeks, our trial subjects saw a significant reduction

CELLULITE BLASTERS

For decades, there have been creams and treatments on the market purporting to cure cellulite. There's little scientific basis for any claims that these topicals actually work. Cellulite is tricky. It's not like regular subcutaneous fat deposits. Instead, fat cells enlarge and push up against the skin, while tough, long cords of connective tissue pull the skin down, creating the dimpled, lumpy effect of an overstuffed mattress. It affects mostly women past the age of puberty and appears on the thighs, buttocks, and stomach. Even with weight loss, it never goes away completely.

But laser and radiofrequency systems are offering some promising solutions. Their underlying technology is similar, and none offer a complete cure, but here are a few that I've tested and found to be the most likely to succeed.

◆ **Cellupulse:** A non-invasive technology that uses sound waves to thin out the layers of fat under the skin. The sound waves increase blood flow as they shock the bodily tissue, in effect shrinking the fat. The treatment was first used on muscles to help patients with sports injuries, and then doctors noticed an interesting side effect—the reduction of cellulite.

◆ **VelaShape:** Also non-invasive, combining bipolar radiofrequency technology with infrared light energy plus vacuum and mechanical massage. It works by contracting and tightening the skin tissue to tone the area and uses suction to increase circulation. Studies have shown a 65 percent reduction in cellulite.

◆ **SmoothShapes:** Uses a combination of laser and light energy, in addition to contoured rollers and a vacuum. The fatty tissue is stimulated with a heated, deep-tissue massage that helps increase circulation to the affected area and tones the skin tissue. The treatment is painless and lasts for approximately 30 minutes. The manufacturer claims the technology not only helps to tone and strengthen the tissues, but can also help reduce water retention. The energy is not as intense as in the VelaShape procedure, but some doctors claim they have seen slightly better results and continual skin improvement up to 6 months after treatment.

◆ **Reaction:** Employs radiofrequency energy to the subcutaneous layers to heat the tissue that contributes to cellulite. The deep heating contributes to the metabolic breakdown of adipocytes—the cells that store fat. It also helps diffuse oxygen in the cells. Again, vacuum therapy aids the treatment by allowing deeper penetration of the energy to the affected areas.

in waist circumference (average 1.5 centimeters, with a quarter of patients losing up to 3 centimeters), and we observed no painful nodules, inflammation, or skin atrophy. This was the fourth clinical study by the company with promising results.

It also helped that our physician who administered the treatments, Dr. Marion Shapiro, has been practicing mesotherapy for years with very consistent results and thousands of happy patients. Dr. Shapiro uses a needle gun with metered doses, spaced 1 inch apart across the treated areas. This ensures that the ingredients get injected evenly and precisely for a perfectly smooth contour. One of our patients, Amanda, recently had the treatment before going on a beach vacation because she wanted to minimize the small lumps of scar tissue and adhesions that remained after her liposuction treatment. She was amazed at how smooth her torso was after just a few treatments. Of course, it's important to bear in mind that mesotherapy is best suited for small areas and body sculpting by contouring smaller areas. This is not a treatment for significant fat debulking.

Mesotherapy is another exciting non-ablative alternative to treating localized fat, and pending the results of these ongoing trials, I believe it's poised to make a global comeback. Nevertheless, I would approach it with extreme caution unless you are fortunate enough to be a patient of Dr. Shapiro's or any other physician who uses well-tested and standardized formulas and has been trained to produce consistent results.

ONE PART OF THE PLAN

Whether it's lipo or Lapex, Zeltiq, or mesotherapy, I am not touting these procedures as replacements for traditional weight loss methods like working out and watching your calorie intake. These fat treatments are not cheap. Depending on which and how many body parts are being targeted, costs can range between $2,000 and $7,000 for any form of lipo, which is a substantial financial outlay. To sustain the results, and for optimum body contouring and skin tightening, it's necessary to stick to a sensible regimen of diet and exercise. You want to be at your healthiest and most fit, otherwise the fat deposits will return—albeit not always in the same place—and you'll lose that perfect body once again.

That being said, no matter how diligent some patients are about following diets, it's not always so easy to get rid of bulging thighs or protruding abdomens past a certain age. And with more than 64 percent of adults either obese or overweight in this country, there will always be a need for this extraordinary technology. The danger comes when patients rely on these treatments too much. These treatments should be only one part of a healthy lifestyle. Too often people get addicted and come back to it when they've gained more weight. They figure if they put on a few extra pounds, there's always lipo. But overuse of procedures like lipo can lead to contour irregularities, and there's also a small risk of scarring from heated nonsurgical treatments.

The ideal body-contouring candidates for any of these procedures are those who take good care of themselves and maintain a relatively healthy weight but still can't budge that small area of protruding tummy fat or love handles. It's for people who see one or two persistent problem areas they'd like to fix, like a saddlebag, flabby upper arms, or cankles. It's not for wholesale debulking. As Americans, we're always looking for the easy solution, but this should not be one of them. Do the hard but gratifying work to keep that body looking young and firm. After undergoing a procedure, many of my patients are inspired to maintain their perfected physique with the healthiest possible lifestyle. They've gotten rid of the fat, and they want it to never come back.

Technology can take you only so far. The rest is up to you.

CHAPTER SIXTEEN

TO CUT OR NOT TO CUT

SCALPELS ARE SO LAST CENTURY

Lipo procedures notwithstanding, most of my patients come to me precisely because they want to avoid surgery. They know I advocate putting off going under the knife for as long as possible—or even better, avoiding it altogether. Unlike the more patient Europeans, we North Americans have been too aggressive about prescribing quick fixes to problems of beauty and aging. We are a microwave culture that wants instant gratification through plastic surgery. But these aren't the best solutions over the long term, and my own patients are beginning to realize it. There's been a strong push-back against the surgical look, especially in the past year. There've been so many sad stories coming out of Hollywood lately that they've turned people off of trying to look like perfect plastic dolls. This is truly the era of the New Natural. Looking "done" is so last century.

When a patient who hasn't followed a strict prevention and maintenance regimen reaches the age of 65 or even 70, the effects of photoaging may be so severe and the gravitational pull so strong that only a surgical procedure can help. But if you follow my tenets from an early age and use the arsenal of minimally invasive technology and cosmeceuticals now available, that day may never come. That's the goal of this book: to help you avoid the knife and look great your whole life.

I believe that as more anti-aging technology hits the mainstream, the number of surgical interventions will drop by at least 50 percent. And age prevention and reversal rejuvenation is a lifetime program even if you have surgery. The aging process is still going on, and if you stop the maintenance programs, you will ultimately go backward in terms of advantages. And a facelift, while dramatic, can only tighten muscles and pull away the skin. It can't give your skin better texture or tone. It won't plump up volume loss. In fact, you will lose volume.

If you are still considering surgery after reading this book, you're going to get two very different opinions, depending on whether you consult a plastic

The Price of Beauty
Cosmetic procedure costs from your twenties to your sixties

IN YOUR TWENTIES

TREATMENT	MONTHLY COST	ANNUAL COST	COST OVER 10 YEARS
Preventive Skin Care—SPF	$25	$300	$3,000
Daily Skin Care/ Antioxidant Regimen	$100	$1,200	$14,400
Acne/Rosacea—Skin Care OTC/Topical	$100	$1,200	$14,400
Acne/Rosacea— Lasers: 1. IPL	$800	$4,000 (x series of 6 treatments)	~$12,000
2. Fraxel for Scars	$1,500	$6,000 (x series of 4–5 treatments)	~$12,000
3. Red/Blue Light	$1,000	$3,000	~$9,000–$12,000

IN YOUR THIRTIES

TREATMENT	MONTHLY COST	ANNUAL COST	COST OVER 10 YEARS
Preventive Skin Care—SPF	$25	$300	$3,000
Daily Skin Care/ Antioxidant Regimen	$100	$1,200	$14,400
Acne/Rosacea—Skin Care OTC/Topical	$100	$1,200	$14,400
Acne/Rosacea— Lasers: 1. IPL	$800	$4,000 (x series of 6 treatments)	~$12,000
2. Fraxel for Scars/Pigment/Fine Lines	$1,500	$6,000 (x series of 4-5 treatments)	~$12,000
3. Red/Blue Light	$1,000	$3,000	~$9,000–$12,000
4. Laser Genesis	$1,200	~$4,800	~$14,400
Anti-Aging Lasers:			
1. IPL (same as above)			
2. Fraxel (same as above)			
3. Laser Genesis (same as above)			
4. Gemini (facial vessels)	$1,500	$1,500	$15,000
5. Thermage Eyes +/or Face	$2,500–$4,000	$2,500–$4,000	$7,500–$12,000
Toxins/Fillers:			
Botox/Dysport (Toxin)	$500–$1,000 (3-4 months)	$500–$1,000	$2,000–$4,000
Juvéderm/Restylane	$800 (once/ twice a year)	$800–$1,600	$8,000–$16,000

surgeon or a dermatologist. Of course a plastic surgeon is going to say you need a face-lift. He or she may be correct depending upon your expectations and the condition of your skin. But I suggest you consult both a surgeon and a dermatologist and then decide. You should hear both sides and be armed with enough information to make the right decision for you. Better yet, go to a practice that has both plastic surgeons and dermatologists, or a practitioner who does both, to get a more balanced opinion.

The reasons we age are universal. We are all subject to genetics and external factors such as photoaging from the sun. We all lose collagen and elasticity,

IN YOUR FORTIES

TREATMENT	MONTHLY COST	ANNUAL COST	COST OVER 10 YEARS
Preventive Skin Care—SPF	$25	$300	$3,000
Daily Skin Care/ Antioxidant Regimen	$100	$1,200	$14,400
Acne/Rosacea— Lasers: 1. IPL	$800	$4,000 (x series of 6 treatments)	~$12,000
2. Fraxel for Scars/Pigment/Fine Lines	$1,500	$6,000 (x series of 4–5 treatments)	~$12,000
3. Laser Genesis	$1,200	~$4,800	~$14,400
Anti-Aging Lasers:			
1. IPL (same as above)			
2. Fraxel (same as above)			
3. Laser Genesis (same as above)			
4. Gemini (facial vessels)	$1,500	$1,500	$15,000
5. Thermage Eyes + Face + Neck	$3,000–$4,500	$2,500–$4,500	$9,000–$13,500
Toxins/Fillers:			
Botox/Dysport (Toxin)	$500–$1,500 (Q 3-4 months)	$1,500–$4,500	$15,000–$45,000
Fillers	$1,600–$2,000 (twice a year)	$3,200–$4,000	$32,000–$40,000

our cells reproduce more slowly, our skin barrier becomes thinner, and the muscle, bone, and fat in the deeper tissues become weaker and less able to support the dermis. And it's all reversible without going under the knife.

I am not saying "never." As a board-certified plastic surgeon, I perform minimally invasive procedures like laser lipolysis and liposuction that involve small incisions. Sometimes gravity takes skin beyond the point where you have the option of a nonsurgical procedure if you want to see dramatic improvement. But less is more. And plastic surgery should be the last resort.

You may have heard the argument that getting a face-lift is cheaper than doing all the natural things it takes to reverse aging and maintain a youthful

IN YOUR FIFTIES TO SIXTIES

TREATMENT	MONTHLY COST	ANNUAL COST	COST OVER 10 YEARS
Preventive Skin Care—SPF	$25	$300	$3,000
Daily Skin Care/ Antioxidant Regimen	$100	$1,200	$14,400
Rosacea— Lasers: 1. IPL	$800	$4,000 (x series of 6 treatments)	~$12,000
2. Laser Genesis	$1,200	~$4,800	~$14,400
Anti-Aging Lasers:			
1. IPL (same as above)			
2. Fraxel for Scars/Pigment/Fine Lines	$1,500	$6,000 (x series of 4-5 treatments)	~$12,000
3. Laser Genesis (same as above)			
4. Gemini (facial vessels)	$1,500	$1,500	$15,000
5. Thermage Eyes + Face + Neck	$3,000–$4,500	$2,500–$4,500	$9,000–$13,500
6. Resurfacing (Fractional or General)	$4,000–$6,000 (once a year)	$4,000–$6,000	$8,000–$12,000
Toxins/Fillers:			
Botox/Dysport (Toxin)	$1,000–$1,500 (Q 3-4 months)	$3,000–$4,500	$30,000–$45,000
Fillers	$1,600–$2,400 (twice a year)	$3,200–$4,800	$32,000–$48,000

look over a lifetime. It's true. The price of a face-lift ranges from $6,000 to $25,000 depending on the location, experience, and reputation of the surgeon and the extent of the surgery itself. As you will see on these pages, the amount you can spend on lasers, Thermage, fillers, and Botox over the years can add up to thousands more dollars. But here's the thing: One face-lift over a lifetime is not going to cut it, if you'll pardon the pun. It will keep things from falling for a decade or so. Then you'll need another and possibly another. And the more you cut, the less natural you will look. You will lose the volume that's vital to a soft, youthful look. And you will still need to spend money on cosmeceuticals and in-office procedures to address issues like skin pigmentation and wrinkles.

One of my patients, Tanya, treated herself to a face-lift when she was 45. She was a singer and felt she needed to take this drastic measure to stay competitive with younger performers and continue to look good onstage. I must admit, the surgeon did a nice job. Tanya paid top dollar for the best, and for a woman her age, she had almost no skin laxity on her neckline, cheeks, or jawline. But by 52, she wasn't looking so fresh anymore. Her skin was much thinner than it was before her face-lift, and the areas around her eyes and mouth were getting crepey. She had beautiful high cheekbones, but her mid-cheek area was getting hollow and she had a gaunt look to her face that was aging her.

Tanya was desperate to avoid that second surgery. She'd seen other women in show business get nipped and tucked one too many times, and she dreaded that artificially pulled look. She came to me to see what could be done to give her back some of the volume she'd lost and to smooth out the texture of her skin. It just so happened that while Tanya was checking in, she saw Peggy, my New Natural poster girl whom you met in Chapter 3.

"Dr. Sadick, whoever did her face, that's what I want. Her skin is amazing!"

"Nobody *did* her, Tanya. That face has never seen a surgeon's knife. And she's over 60. She's been seeing me for years, but the procedures have all been nonsurgical."

"Then tell me what to do and I'll do it."

I immediately put her on an A.M./P.M. regimen of customized skin care to make prevention and renewal a lifetime habit. Then we addressed the texture of her skin with Fraxel to smooth out some of the deeper wrinkles and address the blotchiness caused by sun damage. When that healed, I used Thermage to tighten up some of the little skin laxity there was. Then we addressed volume. Tanya was strikingly beautiful, but there was a hard, angular look to her face that needed softening. I drew some of her blood and spun it down in a centrifuge to extract some platelet-rich plasma, which I then combined with Sculptra volumizing filler, injecting strategically around her midcheek area, under her eyes, along the nasolabial folds, and around her temples. It would be the first of a series of three treatments over 4 months to restore some fullness to Tanya's face and give her skin a glow.

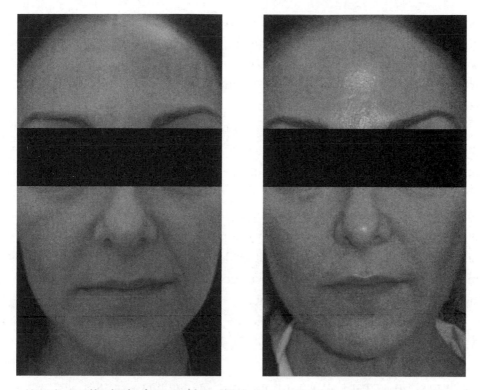

Here is a patient who invested in multiple non-surgical treatments to avoid the surgeon's knife.

It was an expensive recipe of procedures that cost her a little more than $8,000 in the space of 6 months. And I warned Tanya that these treatments would not be a one-shot deal. She needed to be proactive about maintaining what she had. Some of these procedures would need to be repeated every 12 to 18 months if she wanted to keep her skin looking this perfectly refreshed and restored. Throughout her sixth decade, Tanya was looking at an annual beauty bill of $5,000 to $8,000, and the costs would rise the older she got. But for Tanya, it was worth the extra expense. Her stunning looks were a huge part of her professional and personal identity. She'd made a career not only from how she sounded, but from how she looked. She's been coming to me faithfully for 3 years now, and she looks better than she did a decade ago.

If you are experiencing sticker shock right now, I don't blame you. High-end practitioners like me do not come cheap, and it is an unfortunate fact that the best and most cutting-edge procedures are not financially accessible to everyone. My patients typically spend even more than Tanya does—at least $10,000 a year. They can afford it.

But the good news is that even if you do the bare minimum, including the measures you take at home to protect and renew your skin, it will have an impact on how you look decades from now. Good skin care practices, and even the occasional touch-up from Botox and a laser or Thermage treatment every few years, will be of immense benefit in your quest to become your best, most natural-looking self. And the younger you start protecting and maintaining your skin, the less you will need the more expensive, ablative treatments. The way the technology is going, costs may also come down substantially in the decades to come.

Meanwhile, think of it this way: The price of a Grande Skinny Caramel Macchiato at Starbucks is about $4.50. If that or a comparable beverage is your daily indulgence, you are spending $1,642.50 a year and some change (with tax) on a treat that is nothing more than empty calories. That money could have gone toward a course of fillers or paid for at least 18 months' worth of Botox. The average woman spends almost $25,000 on shoes in her lifetime.[24] Think of how many shoes you have in your closet that you never wear. If you spent half that amount, you could afford a decade's worth of laser and Thermage treatments and a lifetime's worth of filler. Radiant skin is far more attractive than a pair of killer heels. And you'll have more closet space. Ladies, you also spend an average of $13,000 on makeup over a lifetime. You wouldn't need to wear half as much if you invested a portion of that money in taking care of your skin. So yes, you may really be able to afford anti-aging treatment. And you are worth every penny.

CHAPTER SEVENTEEN

PUT IT ALL TOGETHER

IT'S NEVER TOO LATE FOR TOTAL RENEWAL

There are no one-size-fits-all anti-aging treatments. Every patient is different, and each deserves state-of-the-art combination approaches to tackle areas of concern safely and gradually. The whole point of successful age reversal is to recognize the individuality of your beauty and custom-build each solution around your particular goals, whether you are striving for age reversal or simply looking to subtly maintain the youthful, healthy skin you already have. Forget the cookie-cutter images you see in Hollywood. That's over. The New Natural ideal is to keep and enhance the beauty you were born with.

This is not about a quick lunchtime lift. Remember, youth is a work in progress. Yes, there are some quick fixes like Botox and filler, but overall it takes commitment to become your best self. You have to be willing to put in some work, too, by protecting and maintaining your skin. The earlier you start the better, but it's never too late for improvement. We can tighten and help strengthen the structures that support the face; we can smooth the skin by ridding it of wrinkles, minimizing pores, and evening out skin tone. We can contour your body and stop hair loss in its tracks. These days, we can do it all. But that doesn't necessarily mean you should. Some treatments may not be appropriate for everyone. As practitioners of aesthetic medicine, it's our job to guide you but ultimately respect your wishes. Total renewal can start with something as small as a light laser peel and a brand-new skin care regimen. At the end of the day, it's what *you* see in the mirror that matters most. The New Natural isn't just about having glowing and gorgeous skin. It's about feeling confident in the skin you're in.

But many of my patients want it all. This is the head-to-toe story of one patient who used just about every nonsurgical weapon in our arsenal, from Fraxel to laser lipolysis, for her total face and body makeover. It was something she'd been wanting to do for herself for a long time. Her name is Brenda, and she's a part-time schoolteacher from northern New Jersey. But let's just call her another poster child for the New Natural:

By my 48th birthday, I wasn't feeling very happy with myself. I'd spent most of my twenties and thirties raising two sons, and now that they were off to college, my husband, Donny, and I were suffering from "empty nest syndrome." It's not that we weren't happy with each other. Our marriage was good. It's just that we'd been so focused on the kids that we forgot to do anything for ourselves. Or rather, I wasn't doing anything for myself. (At least Donny had his golf games.) For so many years I'd identified myself as "Mommy" to everyone: my kids, my students, even Donny. And when I looked in the mirror, that's how I felt: middle-aged and matronly. I needed to get back to the vital woman I knew was still there behind those tired eyes. I just hoped it wasn't too late.

I told Donny how I was feeling. I wanted to make some serious improvements to my appearance—a total head-to-toe makeover, even plastic surgery if it was necessary. Donny always did, and always will, tell me I look beautiful, but I wasn't doing this for him. I didn't need to. This was for me. And luckily we could afford it. Donny still had a well-paid job working as an executive for an insurance company in Manhattan, and over the years I'd managed to put a little money aside from my teaching position. Our boys' college fees were covered through scholarships and their part-time jobs, and our mortgage was totally paid up, so we were more than comfortable. For my birthday gift, Donny offered to pay for most of the work I wanted to have done. "Anything you want, babe," he said. "Just make sure that you go to the best. I don't want some guy talking you into all this plastic surgery you don't need. I want you to look like the woman I married."

I felt the same way. I still wanted to look like me, only better. I did some online research and found Dr. Sadick, and I liked his nonsurgical, natural approach to turning back the clock. I decided to make an appointment at his Park Avenue practice to see what he could do to freshen me up.

Honestly, I was a little intimidated when I sat in his waiting room. The place looked so slick with its white leather sofas and fancy wall murals. Not to mention the other women checking in and out at the reception desk. They were elegant, slim, almost perfect-looking creatures. And a lot of them looked so young! I was starting to feel like I'd come too late. These ladies had obviously been taking great care of themselves their whole lives. I was afraid Dr. Sadick would take one look at me and refer me to some nip/tuck-type plastic surgeon for a total overhaul. When I entered his office, he looked me up and down and smiled that dimpled smile of his.

"What can I do for you, Brenda?"

"Everything, I hope," I said.

My list was a long one. While the texture of my skin was pretty good and I didn't have deep lines, I was starting to get crow's-feet around my eyes, horizontal lines on my forehead, and vertical lines between my eyebrows. Those marionette lines between the outer corners of my mouth and nose were also getting deeper. It made me look sad. And my skin wasn't as firm as it used to be. Not that I had jowls, but I no longer had a nice clean jawline. And my dark circles and eye bags were not cute, either. There was a time when I could get a good night's sleep and they'd disappear. Not so anymore! There's nothing more deflating than having people come up to me and tell me I look tired when I'm not. I liked my mouth, and I wasn't going to be one of those deluded women with blubber lips from too much filler, but I was concerned about some slight feathering above my upper lip, probably from a brief period in my foolish twenties when I smoked and sun-worshipped.

"I see you have a little pigmentation from sun damage, too," said the helpful doc.

Funny, I hadn't noticed until he pointed it out. That must be why my complexion didn't have the glow it used to. I added it to my growing checklist of things I wanted to fix.

Then I moved on to my body. What can I say? After giving birth twice, I never completely got my figure back. I always had nice legs, and they were still more or less intact, but I had cottage cheese on my butt cheeks and a generous muffin top that spilled out over my waistband. My breasts were fine, and I wasn't about to get a boob job—that's where I drew the line. But my middle was squishy and round, and the tops of my arms jiggled to the point where I was wearing long sleeves even on a hot July day.

When I finished running through my laundry list, Dr. Sadick still had that impish grin on his face. In fact, he hadn't even flinched. It was as if he'd already heard my story many times.

"Go ahead and say it, Dr. Sadick. It's too late for me to fix these things without surgery, isn't it?"

"Of course not, Brenda. Everything you want to correct and improve is perfectly suited to a nonsurgical procedure. I am not going to promise you that it will all be easy, painless, or instant. In fact, some of the things you would like to fix could take a few months to see full results. And it will involve multiple treatments and procedures. The total cost is going to run in the thousands. And the results won't be as dramatic as plastic surgery, if that is what you were hoping. This will all add up to you looking like a 5-to-10-year younger and fresher version of yourself. But none of what I am proposing will require cutting or stitching. I promise."

I could tell I'd come to the right place. That was exactly what I wanted to be—a fresher version of myself. He got it.

"Well, Doc, I waited this long to do something myself, so if I have to be a work in progress for the next year, so be it. When do we start?"

We began on the aging issues that were bothering me about my face. Dr. Sadick wanted me to lose a few pounds before we got started on the body-contouring procedures, and I could see his point. I'd only recently started a fitness program, and I still wasn't within 20 pounds of my ideal weight. I needed to do what I could on my own first for the best results, although I didn't have any illusions about ever getting flat abs without a little extra help.

We started with intense pulsed light, or IPL, therapy under a machine called the MedLight C6 to clear my skin of present and future sunspots. I felt some heat and a few pings on my skin, as if I'd been snapped with a rubber band, but overall it was tolerable. I left feeling as though I'd spent a little too much time at the beach. Over the next few days, my skin started to darken and peel, and I felt like a snake shedding its skin. But I did notice a difference once I'd healed. My skin looked brighter. The photofacial even took care of a couple of old acne scars on my fore-head and chin.

A month later, Dr. Sadick went to work on my frown lines with Botox. After a few days, I was thrilled by the dramatic difference a few little shots around my face made. When that settled in, he used filler—Sculptra—all over my face. Sculptra was an appropriate name for this stuff, because it was almost as if he were sculpting my face, filling in areas here and there that needed more volume. I couldn't believe how close he was able to get to my eyes. He filled out the tear troughs and virtually erased my eye bags. I had to go through three treatments spaced a few weeks apart, but at the end of 3 months, when all that filler settled in, my skin was smooth and glowing, and most of the wrinkles were gone. There was also a creamy, baby soft texture to my skin that I had not felt in years.

My eyes still needed more work. While they were already looking much better, the skin immediately under my eyes was still crepey, and my upper lids were starting to droop. Dr. Sadick decided to use two high-tech procedures—Fraxel re:pair and Thermage—to correct these problems. The purpose of the Fraxel was to resurface the skin below my eyes and tighten a little. The treatment did sting somewhat, and I couldn't leave the house without sunglasses for about a week and a half afterward, but the end result looked spectacular. I looked as though I'd had a year's worth of beauty rest. Then we used Thermage on my face, neck, and upper eyelids to tighten. It took a while to kick in. The procedure wasn't fun, and I had my doubts about how much tightening I could get, but after 2 months I began to notice how much more open my eyes looked, and after 6 months my sagging lids were a distant memory. Overall, the effect on my face was more subtle, but when I look at pictures of myself before the procedure, I can see the skin on my cheeks and jowls is much firmer.

I asked Dr. Sadick why he couldn't have just used the Fraxel over my whole face and skipped the IPL procedure. It seemed redundant to me to use two different technologies. But he explained that he believed in matching the right treatment to the problem. Apart from my eyes, the lines and pigment on my face were minor and did not require a more aggressive procedure like Fraxel. Why increase the downtime and risk of injury? Whatever the reasoning, the cumulative effect of all these procedures was peeling back the years layer by layer. No one noticed anything dramatic, because the process was so gradual, but friends I hadn't seen in a few months were looking at me sideways. I didn't mind one bit.

While my face was a work in progress, I got to work on my body. I gave myself 6 months to get in the best shape I could. The confidence boost I got from each little cosmetic improvement energized me. I joined a yoga class twice a week and did weights and resistance exercise with a personal trainer three times a week. I also cut back on the sodas and carbs. It wasn't a crash diet. I wanted to reach a level I could maintain so my body-contouring procedures would hold. I lost 15 pounds and reached my weight goal. A nice side effect of this weight loss was that my cellulite went away. But I still had a few stubborn problem areas I wanted to treat: my pooch and obliques, the pocket of fat at the backs of my upper arms, and the tops of my inner thighs where the skin always chafed.

When I saw Dr. Sadick again, he was pleased with how far I had come with my diet and exercise program. He said I'd be a great candidate for laser lipolysis. All I needed was a local anesthetic. I might be a little sore afterward, and I'd have to wear compression bandages for a week, but I could be back at work the next day. That was fine with me. There was something satisfying about the whirr and suction noise of the machine extracting my fat. The pain was minimal, or maybe I was too excited to notice. I was finally getting rid of the unsightly flab I didn't like my husband to see. A few weeks later, when the swelling had gone down, I had a waist! I was so proud of my new body. I'd lost three dress sizes and had the perfect excuse to buy a new wardrobe. Donny couldn't take his eyes off me. We even made love with the lights on!

The total bill for all of this was breathtaking, as I had been warned: close to $15,000! I'm almost ashamed to admit that I could spend that much money on my appearance. On the other hand, I'd been putting my own needs on a back burner for the past two decades, and if this was what it took to bring back the old Brenda, it was money well spent. And it's not the last of it. I've learned that protecting my investment and maintaining these face and body improvements will continue to cost. Dr. Sadick put me on a custom-designed skin care regimen. And to sustain the effect of the Sculptra, I have to plan on going back every couple of years. I'll need more Botox every few months, and it wouldn't hurt to redo the Thermage every year or two.

I feel privileged that I am able to afford this. I know it's not within everyone's means. It's given me so much confidence and drive. I'm like the Energizer Bunny. I feel healthier. I socialize more. I'm branching out in my teaching career and doing some consulting on the side. I'm even taking up golf so I can spend more time with Donny on weekends. And I'm *happy!* This was a total makeover, inside and out. So I can't really put a price on what Dr. Sadick did for me. He gave me back the natural beauty I was born with, and then some.

ABOUT THE
AUTHOR

Some people call him a mad scientist. Others call him eccentric, even evangelistic. But to his many thousands of patients, he is a genius.

Considered by his peers to be one of the world's leading dermatologists, Dr. Neil Sadick is a widely acknowledged expert on aging and a pioneer in the fields of minimally invasive and non-invasive aesthetic surgery. Founder of the Sadick Research Group, Dr. Sadick has a thriving Park Avenue practice where he offers patients the full spectrum of anti-aging and skin rejuvenation treatments using the very latest in proven technologies.

Unlike some of his colleagues, who simply buy the machines without fully understanding how they work or how to use them, this ingenious innovator has a direct hand in developing much of what is new and revolutionary in the science of beauty. Dr. Sadick has the ability to understand not only the ins and outs of the technology we use, but also how it can complement other treatments and take on new roles to push the frontiers of skin health. Not content simply to apply the new treatments, he learns how they work and how they interact with the human body, to continually improve their efficacy, comfort, and safety. He then collaborates with companies to fine-tune their treatment protocols and continually challenges them to provide new and more effective treatment options.

A member of the board of trustees for the Dermatology Foundation, clinical professor of dermatology at Weill Cornell Medical College in New York City, and past president of the Cosmetic Surgery Foundation, Dr. Sadick also serves as the global medical advisor to Christian Dior, where he assists the company in developing breakthrough skin care products. As a physician with extensive experience in multiple specialties, including internal medicine, cosmetic surgery, dermatology, phlebology, and hair transplant surgery, Dr. Sadick has documented his seminal research in hundreds of scientific articles, books, and papers. The best skin doctors know that if it's new and it works, somehow, some way, Dr. Sadick had a hand in its development.

Named a "Best Doctor" multiple times by *New York* magazine, the author has been at the forefront of two of the most talked-about new alternatives in the treatment of aging—non-ablative lasers and the newest injectable wrinkle "fillers." Dr. Sadick, whose clinical trials contributed to FDA approvals in both areas, has been working with lasers since the 1980s. He helped pioneer the first intense pulsed light treatment systems. When he said lasers could be used for hair removal, skin tightening, and body shaping, his colleagues said he was crazy. All three are now standard treatments. When he saw the possibilities that fillers held for smoothing wrinkles, building volume, and stimulating new collagen, he was again laughed at, but 20 years later fillers have become the gold standard in the dermatologist's office.

Dr. Sadick came to this field through his love of science. The New York native was a gifted child who studied at the renowned Stuyvesant High School. His early passions for sports, gadgets, and all things scientific eventually morphed into a determination to become a doctor. Dr. Sadick studied internal medicine and soon switched to dermatology. The appeal was the way it merges disciplines and requires a multifaceted use of his skills. Dr. Sadick saw how he could combine his extensive knowledge of how internal health manifests on the surface of the skin with the dexterity of his hands. The doctor's talent, along with an unerring naturalistic aesthetic sense, makes him one of the most sought-after cosmetic surgeons in the country. His unusual combination of gifts allows him to gracefully transform patients into younger, better versions of themselves and, often, save lives. Many patients seek out Dr. Sadick after other doctors fail to diagnose potentially lethal causes of skin lesions and rashes. They fly in from around the country to find medical solutions for hair loss that stumped legions of specialists, only to learn they have underlying hormonal conditions that are easily treatable. His mission is as much about health as it is about beauty.

There are dozens of celebrity doctors out there, but unlike Dr. Sadick, they don't go past the surface. They're the ones more interested in quick fixes. But you don't have to look far to see how their methods are flawed. Their own features are as waxlike and frozen as the faces of their poor misguided patients.

Dr. Sadick's low-key style belies his status as the world's leading proponent of anti-aging science and technology. He is trusted by the world's most beautiful celebrities, but you wouldn't know they were his patients. Unlike many plastic surgeons and dermatologists, he doesn't put his personal stamp on these women and make them look "done." No one would ever guess which doctor has had a hand in these flawless faces, because their look is completely natural and individual. These are the stars in their prime who look better and better with each passing year, yet no one can quite figure out how. They continue to look gorgeous but still natural, and that, along with ensuring the ease of his patients, is the key to his whole approach. He is continually experimenting, refining, innovating. He has propelled the evolution of the most popular dermatological advancements available, but he won't rest until he has explored and adapted all that's new and miraculous in dermatology. It's his unrelenting mission to make the future of age reversal a reality today.

ACKNOWLEDGMENTS

A heartfelt thanks to all of my loyal patients over the past 30 years. It is because of you that I strive to be more. To my dedicated and hard-working staff at Sadick Dermatology, for all that you do. A very special thanks to my Chief Operating Officer, Adam Dinkes, who has been instrumental in our success and whose sharp eye and devotion to detail was a godsend in producing this book. A special mention also to Jackie Toma and Laura and Diana Palmisano for their invaluable input, and to Samantha Marshall, for "translating" this scientist in a way that's accessible to all. To Carol Mann, my tireless literary agent, and my excellent editors at Rodale, Pam Krauss and Victoria Glerum. It's a distinct pleasure to work with the best. Finally, to all the doctors and academics who are continually raising the bar in the field of dermatology and making beautiful, healthy, and natural-looking skin a reality for patients at any age.

REFERENCES

1 (page 10)

Aesthetic Medicine News, "Study Reveals What Women Want When Considering Aesthetic Procedures," http://www.aestheticmedicinenews.com/study-reveals-what-women-want-when-considering-aesthetic-procedures.htm

2 (page 15)

See: Centers for Disease Control and Prevention, "Skin Cancer Statistics," http://www.cdc.gov/cancer/skin/statistics/

American Academy of Dermatology, "Sunscreens," http://www.aad.org/media-resources/stats-and-facts/prevention-and-care/sunscreens

Skin Cancer Foundation, "Skin Cancer Facts," http://www.skincancer.org/Skin-Cancer-Facts/

Skin Cancer Foundation, "Guidelines," http://www.skincancer.org/nonmelanoma-skin-cancer-incidence-jumps-by-over-300-percent.html

3 (page 21)

Journal of Cosmetic Laser Therapy, June 2010; Vol. 12, Issue 3: pp 157–62

4 (page 30)

Rosacea Review, Spring 2004

5 (page 32)

Archives of Dermatology, May 2007; Vol. 143, No. 5: pp 606–12

6 (page 73)

Pauling, L: *How To Live Longer and Feel Better* (New York: WH Freeman and Company, 1986), 89–91

7 (page 74)

Journal of the American Academy of Dermatology, June 2003, Vol. 48: pp. 866–74

8 (page 116)

Sadick Dermatology, "Veins," http://www.sadickdermatology.com/veins.html

9 (page 117)

Sadick Dermatology, "Veins," http://www.sadickdermatology.com/veins.html

10 (page 150)

McKinsey Quarterly, May 2008

11 (page 154)

Morello, D.C., Colon, G.A., Fredericks, S., Iverson, R., Singer, R. "Patient safety in accredited office surgical facilities." *Plastic and Reconstructive Surgery* 99: 1496, 1997

12 (page 155)

From Patient Experiences, Perceptions and Attitudes on Post-surgical Side Effects and Complications, by Harris Interactive for the American Society of Plastic Surgeons and Merck & Co

13 (page 163)

American Society for Aesthetic Plastic Surgery, "2007 Statistics," http://www.surgery.org/press/statistics-2007.php

14 (page 166)
   Archives of Dermatology, Feb. 2007; Vol. 143, No. 2: pp 155–63

15 (page 184)
   Neil S. Sadick and Donald Charles Richardson, *Your Hair: Helping to Keep It: Treatment and Prevention of Hair Loss for Men and Women*, (Yonkers: Consumer Reports Books, 1992)

16 (page 185)
   Journal of the American Academy of Dermatology, Aug. 2010, Vol. 63: pp 252–58

17 (page 191)
   University of Pennsylvania School of Medicine News, May 16, 2007; see also: http://www/uphs.upenn.edu/News-Releases/May07/hair-follicles-regeneration.html

18 (page 192)
   Histogen Corporate Website, "HSC Trial Shows Continued Significant Hair Growth at One Year Follow-Up," April 13, 2010

19 (page 198)
   Cosmetic Surgery Times, May 2009

20 (page 204)
   PlasticSurgeryResearch.info, "Cosmetic Plastic Surgery Research: Statistics and Trends for 2001–2007," http://cosmeticplasticsurgerystatistics.com/statistics.html

21 (page 204)
   http://cosmeticplasticsurgerystatistics.com/statistics.html

22 (page 208)
   Aesthetic Surgery Journal, July/August 2010 Vol. 30, No. 4, pp: 593–602; see also: http://aes.sagepub.com/content/30/4/593.abstract

23 (page 211)
   Journal of Dermatologic Surgery, April 2006; Vol. 32, No. 4: pp 465–80

24 (page 222)
   Gocompare.com survey first published in the *Daily Express*, U.K., April 18, 2010, http://dailyexpress.co.uk/posts/view/183444/women-s-16k-shoe-bill

INDEX

Boldface page references indicate illustrations. <u>Underscored</u> references indicate boxed text.